Published by RMU Press, Highland, Michigan.
Layout and cover artwork by Gysèle Maas, Boston, Massachusetts.

RMU Press also publishes this book in a variety of electronic formats. Some content that appears in print may not be available in electronic books. For more information, visit the companion website at theMUguide.com.

For information about special discounts for bulk purchases, please send a request to **info@theMUguide.com**.

ISBN: 978-0615750705

Printed in the United States of America

FIRST EDITION 10 9 8 7 6 5 4 3 2 1

Jonathon L. Dreyer

Keith J. Dreyer, *DO, PhD, FACR, FSIIM*

MEANINGFUL USE ESSENTIALS

Your **First 2 Years**

“...To improve the quality of our health care while lowering its cost, we will make the immediate investments necessary to ensure that within five years, all of America's medical records are computerized. This will cut waste, eliminate red tape, and reduce the need to repeat expensive medical tests. But it just won't save billions of dollars and thousands of jobs—it will save lives by reducing the deadly but preventable medical errors that pervade our healthcare system...”

President Barack Obama
Speech on the Economy
George Mason University, Fairfax, VA
January 8, 2009

Contents

Part I:

Part II:

Part III:

Introduction

With billions of dollars in available incentive payments for eligible professionals in the United States, every physician has the opportunity to receive up to $44,000 for achieving meaningful use before 2015. But in order to receive all incentive payments, meaningful use must begin by 2012. And starting in 2015, Medicare payment reductions will begin for not demonstrating meaningful use—hundreds of millions of dollars are at risk annually, and that number may reach billions if private payers start to mirror federal guidelines.

What is meaningful use?

Meaningful use, a term born out of the American Recovery and Reinvestment Act (ARRA) of 2009, refers to the use of certified electronic health record technology (CEHRT; pronounced "cert") to promote health care improvements and advance the electronic exchange of information among health care professionals. This program, designed to encourage health care professionals and hospitals to use CEHRT and demonstrate compliance through a series of measures and criteria, provides financial incentives for achieving health and efficiency goals over a prescribed timeframe.

Who is this guide for?

Everyone involved in the management and delivery of medical services—ranging from physicians to practice administrators, IT leads and CIOs, to healthcare IT vendors, and others. This guide primarily focuses on the Medicare version of the program for eligible professionals (EPs) and will help you develop, execute, and maintain your MU strategy.

Inside this Essential Series guide

This guide is divided into three parts, each of which focuses on core components of Stage 1 Meaningful Use, objectives and measures relevant to your first two years of participation, and workload reduction considerations for medical professionals.

- **Part I** takes a detailed look at the criteria that makes up Stage 1 Meaningful Use and provides a systematic approach to presenting key program requirements, offering workload reduction considerations and practice-level policy guidance, breaking down functional tasks, and outlining attestation specifications.
- **Part II** moves beyond Stage 1 and examines Stage 2 Meaningful Use and the impact the Stage 2 Final Rules have on Stage 1 of the program.
- **Part III** provides a compilation of useful FAQs as well as a variety of tools and resources to help you during your first two years of meaningful use and beyond.

Online companion

Meaningful use is an evolving concept, and new information is always being published. The companion website to this guide, **theMUguide.com**, offers notification of content changes and information updates to be used in conjunction with this book and other guides in the series.

Quick Response (QR) codes and direct URLs

To enhance your experience, we have incorporated QR codes and direct URLs throughout the text of this guide. These codes will direct you to the online companion website where the most up-to-date information can be found. In order to use the QR codes, you will need a smartphone with a camera and QR code software. There are a number of free QR readers available, including Red Laser, QuickMark, and ScanLife, for multiple mobile device platforms.

MU Overview

A five-year promise

On January 24, 2009, during his first Weekly Address as 44th president of the United States, President Barack Obama said that the nation's health records will be computerized within five years in order to lower health care costs, cut medical errors, and improve care.

In an effort to entice health care providers to jump onboard and begin to computerize their records, the government is incentivizing eligible physicians and hospitals under the Centers for Medicare and Medicaid Services (CMS) Electronic Health Records (EHR) Incentive Programs: paying up to $44,000 under Medicare and $63,750 under Medicaid. However, there is a catch. In order to qualify for this funding, provisions of the American Recovery and Reinvestment Act of 2009 and the Health Information Technology for Economic and Clinical Health (HITECH) Act require health care providers to show they are "meaningful users" of "certified" electronic health record systems over a specific timeline.

The road ahead

There is considerable pressure for all physicians to become meaningful users under the CMS EHR Incentive Programs. Determining provider eligibility, evaluating certified technology, and reviewing IT infrastructure are just a few of the necessary components for successful participation in these government programs. Meaningful use is moving rapidly, but the program is following a clear trajectory. Stage 1 Meaningful Use focuses on electronic data capture, while Stages 2 and 3 expand on this foundation by promoting quality, structured information exchange, safety, efficiency, and population health improvements.

The practice of medicine is changing, and EHR technology will undoubtedly provide medical providers with more information than ever before. Health care professionals will be able to access increased information about patients, share that information with colleagues at other facilities, and improve the quality of individual patients' care while monitoring and reporting data to federal committees to achieve health improvements for the population as a whole.

Goals of meaningful use

By focusing on the effective use of EHRs with certain capabilities, the HITECH Act makes it clear that the adoption of records is not a goal in itself: it is the use of EHRs to achieve health and efficiency goals that matters. HITECH's incentives and assistance programs seek to improve the health of Americans and the performance of their healthcare system through the meaningful use of EHRs to achieve five primary health care goals:

- Improve quality, safety, and efficiency while reducing health disparities.
- Engage patients and families in their health care.
- Promote and improve public and population health.
- Improve care coordination between providers.
- Ensure adequate privacy and security protections for personal health information.

In the context of the EHR Incentive Programs, demonstrating meaningful use is the key to receiving the incentive payments. It requires meeting a series of objectives that makes use of EHRs potential and is related to the improvement of quality, efficiency, and patient safety in the healthcare system through the use of certified technology.

10 Steps to Meaningful Use

Prepare

STEP 1: Understanding the fundamentals of meaningful use
STEP 2: Determining your eligibility and financial impact of the program
STEP 3: Determining your meaningful use measure requirements

Develop

STEP 4: Meeting with your practice stakeholders
STEP 5: Meeting with your IT vendors

Execute

STEP 6: Planning your meaningful use technological and operational strategies
STEP 7: Acquiring and implementing certified EHR technology

Sustain

STEP 8: Registering online with CMS
STEP 9: Monitoring your meaningful use compliance regularly
STEP 10: Attesting online with CMS

Below, we outline a proven 10-step strategy for EPs to follow as they approach meaningful use—preparing, developing, executing, and sustaining a strategy for success. First, we start with preparation, including a review of meaningful use fundamentals, eligibility requirements, and the financial impact of this government program. After that, we move on to developing your strategy through practice stakeholder meetings and discussions with IT vendors. Next, we focus on execution of your strategy through technical and operational planning as well as acquiring and implementing new certified technology, if needed. Finally, we consider ways to sustain meaningful use including program registration, compliance-monitoring using dashboards and scorecards, and attesting with CMS.

Prepare

In this first section of the 10-step approach to achieving meaningful use, we discuss recommendations for understanding program fundamentals, determining your eligibility, assessing the financial impact, and determining your meaningful use measure requirements.

Step 1: Understanding the fundamentals of meaningful use

Meaningful use success begins with understanding the fundamentals. Whether that means visiting the government program website, going to lectures, reading articles, listening to podcasts, attending tradeshows, or reading the nearly one thousand pages of regulations, it is imperative that you understand the fundamentals of the CMS EHR Incentive Programs and what they mean to your practice.

Step 2: Determining your eligibility and financial impact

It is recommended that you review your own practice setting and group billing history to determine your eligibility for the incentive program and conduct a meaningful use analysis using your group's practice and individual EP data.

Preparing an analysis before developing your strategy not only helps you to better understand the impact of the Medicare EHR Incentive Program on your practice, but also provides a baseline for internal and external meaningful use discussions and planning. Fortunately, there are tools available online to assist with this process (for example, **www.DoYouMU.com**). In order to complete your online analysis, you must answer the following questions:

- How many physicians practice in your group?
- What is your total CMS revenue?
- Are you part of a multi-specialty practice?
- Does your practice plan to enroll and participate in the CMS EHR Incentive Programs?
- When do you plan to begin meaningful use of certified technology?
- What percentage of your CMS volume is Inpatient Hospital (POS21)?
- What percentage of your CMS volume is Emergency Room (POS23)?
- Does your group practice in a Health Professional Shortage Area (HPSA)?

What if you are eligible for both versions? EPs who are eligible for both the Medicare and Medicaid EHR Incentive Programs must choose which incentive program they wish to participate in when they register. Before 2015, any EP may switch programs only once after the first incentive payment is initiated.

Step 3: Determining your meaningful use measure requirements

In conjunction with determining your eligibility and financial impact, you should also analyze your practice to determine your meaningful use measure requirements and exclusion opportunities. As we've already discussed, the incentive program is based on individual EPs, so all physicians at your practice may not have the same requirements. For example, if you have a group of 10 physicians, you really have to look at each physician to determine their individual exclusion opportunities.

This assessment of your practice will prove invaluable in determining which of the objectives and measures of the Medicare EHR Incentive Program your practice will need to perform and demonstrate in order to achieve meaningful use. Your group may be able to claim exclusions for several of the measures based on individual EPs meeting exclusion criteria.

Remember, you will need to perform an analysis for each EP in your practice in order to fully determine the final set of core and menu set objectives and measures required to achieve meaningful use.

Develop

In the second section of the 10-step approach to achieving meaningful use, we discuss techniques for developing your strategy by meeting with your practice stakeholders and IT vendors.

Step 4: Meeting with your practice stakeholders

A key step on your path to achieving meaningful use involves not only an analysis of your existing IT environment, but also meeting with the meaningful use stakeholders at your organization. Conducting an infrastructure analysis and working with others at your practice will ensure you have the necessary plans in place to be successful on your journey toward meaningful use. Identify your practice stakeholders and determine if a meaningful use taskforce exists at an institutional level within your organization. If you practice in a hospital setting and a taskforce exists, it is recommended that a representative from your practice join that group.

- **Hospital Setting:** It is important for you to understand your institutional plan. If you practice in a hospital setting, it is essential for you to speak with your CIO, CMIO, and any other key individuals that are responsible for meaningful use. You may discover that your EPs are able to leverage your organization's certified EHR technology to achieve meaningful use.
- **Group Practice Setting:** If you work predominately in a group practice setting, speak with your medical director to determine if your group will be participating in the CMS EHR Incentive Programs. Based on this discussion, you will need to ensure that your practice has the appropriate mix of certified EHR technology to satisfy all meaningful use measures and objectives.

Consider your practice setting as part of your plan for determining potential solution options. Identifying your patient mix as well as practice scenario allows you to better understand the implications of meaningful use on your individual EPs and group.

Building your meaningful use team

If your group is large, you will want to build a series of meaningful use sub-teams and designate a lead for each functional area. If you are at a smaller practice, it is likely that a small handful of individuals will share these responsibilities. Either way, your core team should schedule routine meetings and develop a clear path with tangible goals and outcomes in mind.

The **MU Taskforce Core Team** should provide oversight for all of your practice's meaningful use-related initiatives. For hospital-based practices, this includes participation in facility-wide meaningful use meetings and planning with your organization's core initiatives team. Within your core team, you should consider implementing a plan and creating sub-teams with defined responsibilities.

- **Project Management Team**
  - Develop, implement, and monitor your practice's meaningful use plan.
  - Communicate with IT vendors on technology, certification, reporting, and attestation.
  - Create meaningful use educational materials for EPs, manage upgrades, implementations, and timelines with IT vendors.

- **Financial Analysis Team**
  - Calculate financial impact of meaningful use and make recommendations.
  - Track future stages and financial impact.
  - Monitor projections and incentive payments against plan.

- **EP Support Team**
  - Evaluate and monitor provider readiness.
  - Work with project management team and reporting and compliance team to formalize and deliver an education program to EPs.
  - Act as liaison between EPs and the core team.

- **Privacy and Security Team**
  - Monitor meaningful use requirements and make recommendations.
  - Develop and implement a plan to meet requirements.

- **Reporting and Compliance Team**
  - Create plan for achieving, demonstrating, and reporting meaningful use requirements.
  - Develop reports for EPs.
  - Maintain and sustain program compliance.
  - Contribute to education plan.

Taking the time to plan your strategy and leverage the work being done by others within your organization will enable you to meet all of your meaningful use goals. Collaborating with decision-makers and key users will ensure an easier transition toward meaningful use compliance.

Step 5: Meeting with your IT vendors

Once you've met with your practice stakeholders and fully understand the meaningful use plans of your organization, you will be ready to meet with your existing IT vendors and the potential IT partners that will help you achieve meaningful use and meet the technological requirements of the program for which your EPs have enrolled.

Seeking the ideal IT vendor partner

Partnering with the right technology provider is critical to the success of your meaningful use project. Seek a technology partner that is committed to providing not only solutions that are certified for the CMS EHR Incentive Programs, but also ones that provide guidance and support to help your organization recognize the impact of the program and better understand what you need to do to successfully roll out your meaningful use strategy.

If you are in the market to replace or upgrade your existing IT infrastructure, you should seek an IT partner who supports your meaningful use strategy by:

- **Extending a commitment to meaningful use.** Pursue working with an IT solution vendor that is committed to driving the effort toward meaningful use for all of their clients—select a technology provider that understands the value of meaningful use and is dedicated to assisting their customers in satisfying objectives of the government program and maintain compliance with the evolving meaningful use criteria.
- **Demonstrating a clear path to meeting meaningful use objectives.** This includes finding a partner with a clear road map that outlines a detailed plan for certification including timelines and a list

of meaningful use criteria they plan to satisfy with their solutions. The ideal partner should also have clear plans for accommodating future program changes and future program requirements.

- **Simplifying processes by offering a dedicated services team to support the technology.** Engaging with a software provider that is educated on the topic of meaningful use is key. The optimal partner should have experience in assisting clients understand, apply for, and successfully demonstrate meaningful use of certified EHR technology. They should be agile and have a proactive plan in place to provide continued support and updates as federal regulations evolve.
- **Providing flexibility to integrate certified solutions with existing technology and workflows.** Seek a provider that offers flexible solutions to provide minimal impact and disruption to your existing workflows. This includes integrating the technology with your existing solutions and providing effective communication with other systems.

Meaningful use is a long-term strategy and the ideal IT provider is one that you can develop a "true" partnership with to ensure alignment with your meaningful use goals and objectives. Taking the time to evaluate your solution providers and their technology will be instrumental to your success with the program.

Execute

In this third section of the 10-step approach to achieving meaningful use, we discuss techniques for executing your strategy through planning your technological and operational strategies and acquiring and implementing certified technology.

Step 6: Planning your meaningful use technological and operational strategies

The steps leading up to your operational planning will probably not require outside assistance. However, this is the point in the 10-step approach that you begin to spend money and implement your strategy, and it is also the point at which your existing workflow and processes may potentially be impacted. As a result, Step 6 is the first time in the process that it may be appropriate to seek consultative assistance.

There are a number of meaningful use consultants in the field ranging from full-service agencies to smaller, specialized meaningful use consulting service providers. Many of these consulting firms offer services that help align your performance improvement objectives with your technical and operational goals. Consultative assistance can be beneficial for budget preparation, workflow documentation, technical specifications and analysis, connectivity and data exchange, defining vendor and technology requirements, and reviewing your existing IT infrastructure.

In addition to consultants, Regional Extension Centers (RECs) have been established to help EPs as they tackle meaningful use. While the RECs target their assistance to eligible primary care providers in smaller practices, they also serve as resources for all providers in a given geographic region. For the full list of RECs, go to **recs.theMUguide.com**.

Whether you decide to use outside services, an REC, or plan your technological and operational strategy internally, the key objective of your planning efforts should be to minimize EP workflow burden. You will need to determine how much technology is required to make certain that your EPs do not have to perform unnecessary duplicate entry or redundant data capture.

Allocating resources and clearly defining clinical and administrative staff responsibilities for meaningful use will be critical to your success. Leveraging your care team, practice staff, informatics leads, administrators, and your EPs will be instrumental in planning and implementing the various aspects of your meaningful use operational and technical strategy.

Step 7: Acquiring and implementing certified EHR technology

Once you have determined your operational and technological requirements, you may need to acquire or implement certified EHR technology to comply with program requirements not satisfied by your existing technology. This involves considering potential upgrades or add-ons to your EMR, practice management system, and any other IT platform that may be used to demonstrate meaningful use. Also, it is important that your practice has access to a meaningful use dashboard so that your group can view and track all of your individual EP meaningful use measures to ensure ongoing compliance. This functionality might be provided by one of your existing systems or may require implementation of a separate dashboard application.

Since you have to monitor each EP separately, and have so many measures to keep track of, you will need a central system to monitor all of your EP activity, across all patients, for each physician in your practice. A dashboard allows your senior administrators or individual EPs to check their compliance status for a given attestation period. It also provides a record of individual EP activity, which may prove helpful in the event of an audit.

As part of building your technology acquisition and upgrade plan, you will need to conduct product certification status checks. Don't forget that product certification is specific to both a vendor's product and its specific version. In other words, you may need to upgrade your technology to a newer version of software from your IT vendor in order to meet the certified EHR technology requirement.

It's at this stage that the Certified HIT Product List (CHPL) is an excellent resource for searching CEHRT by product name, vendor name, CHPL number (if known) or specific certification criteria met. This authoritative and comprehensive listing of certified Complete EHRs and EHR Modules offers a certification summary bar and shopping cart to aid in your certified technology search. To view the full list of CEHRT, go to **chpl.theMUguide.com**.

Sustain

In this fourth and final section of the 10-step approach to achieving meaningful use for EPs, we discuss the requirements for sustaining your strategy through online registration with CMS, regular compliance monitoring, and the reporting period attestation process.

Step 8: Registering online with CMS

Once you've determined your practice's eligibility for the CMS EHR Incentive Programs, each EP will need to register online using the Medicare and Medicaid EHR Incentive Programs Registration and Attestation System. Registration must be completed prior to submitting meaningful use attestation. Even though registration and attestation can occur at the same time, it is advisable not to wait until your practice is ready to attest to register for the program. While an EP can register prior to possessing all necessary certified EHR technology, this information is required before an EP can attest.

All EPs applying under the Medicare version of the program are required to have a National Provider Identifier (NPI) and National Plan and Provider Enumeration System (NPPES) account. All EPs will also need to be enrolled in the Provider Enrollment, Chain and Ownership System (PECOS). You can check the enrollment status of an EP, and if needed, enroll in the system, via the CMS EHR Incentive Programs website.

CMS also allows EPs to designate a third party to register and attest on their behalf. If an EP or practice chooses to do so, the individuals performing these tasks will need to have an Identity and Access Management System (I&A) account and must be associated with each EP and their NPI. If the user working on behalf of your EPs does not have an account, one can be obtained via the I&A Security Check on the program's official website.

MU Registration Process

The meaningful use program registration process for EPs is straight-forward and on average takes fifteen to twenty minutes per EP. Once an EP has all of the required accounts setup, they must complete a three-piece questionnaire to successfully register for the program.

- First, the EP will be required to select the version of the program for which they are applying. EPs that are eligible for both versions of the program must choose which incentive program they wish to participate in at this point. Before 2015, an EP may switch programs only once after the first incentive payment is issued.
- Next, the EP will need to select their physician type.
- The initial registration survey also asks if the registering EP is currently using a certified EHR and to supply the certified EHR number. While this is not a mandatory requirement for registration, the EP will need to provide this information prior to submitting attestation.
- EP name and identifier information is recorded under personal information and is automatically retrieved from the EP's NPI record. At this stage, an EP must also choose the Payee TIN Type. If the payments are to be sent to the EP directly, they will choose the SSN option. If the payments should be sent to a practice or group associated with the EP, the EIN option will be selected. Based on selection, additional details may be required.
- Like the EP's personal information, the practice address and contact details associated with the EP will be automatically populated from the NPI record.
- Once this information is entered, the EP will have an opportunity to verify their registration submission. After verifying that all of the information is correct, the EP must review and agree to a legal notice before their registration can be submitted.
- Once the disclaimer is accepted, the registration website will notify the EP of successful registration if the registration passes all validations. Since the EP will not receive an email confirmation, the EP should record their registration ID and print a copy of the submission receipt page.

Step 9: Monitoring your meaningful use compliance regularly

Once you have your meaningful use infrastructure up and running, you will need to regularly monitor your compliance against each individual EP's incentive program requirements. This includes implementing a tracking mechanism or dashboard and monitoring the individual EP and group level statuses.

The supplier of your certified EHR technology will provide compliance dashboards for your group. At a minimum, the dashboards that you implement for meaningful use will need to track and allow for reporting by individual EP, facility/location, and date range as well as numerator and denominator for those measures that require such information be reported. It is important to possess a dashboard that generates this data in a format that provides all pertinent information required for attestation. Keep in mind that you will need to track compliance for each individual EP in your practice group.

In year one, EPs are only required to report ninety days of data, but if an EP fails even one measure, they will have to begin the ninety-day period for attestation again. As this process will be new to your practice, it is recommended that you monitor your EP compliance on a daily basis so that you have ample time to correct any issues should they arise. Keep these tips in mind as you plan for and approach the attestation process.

Step 10: Attesting online with CMS

Attestation, or the process of legally stating to CMS that an EP has demonstrated meaningful use of certified EHR technology, is the final step in our 10-step process. Attestation is conducted using the same system that is used for registration—the Medicare and Medicaid EHR Incentive Programs Registration and Attestation System. Prior to attesting as an EP under the Medicare program, you will need to have:

- Determined your eligibility to participate in the Medicare program.
- Successfully registered for the Medicare program on the CMS EHR Incentive Programs Registration System.

- Met the required number of core set, menu set, and clinical quality measures.
- Recorded meeting your meaningful use criteria for the appropriate time period.

MU Attestation Process

Similar in look and feel to the registration pages, the attestation process guides the EP or designated third party through a series of topics including attestation information, core measures, menu measures, core CQMs, alternate core CQMs, and discretionary CQMs. The attestation process is as follows:

- First, the EP will need to provide basic attestation information to begin the process. This includes an EHR Certification Number, reporting period start date and reporting period end date. For the first year, the reporting period must be a minimum of ninety consecutive days. For each subsequent year, the attestation period must be 365 days (or 366 in a leap year like 2012). It is important to note that the CMS EHR Certification Number (which is 15 alphanumeric characters) is different than the ONC CHPL Product Number issued to the EP's technology provider.
- Next, the EP will need to complete all questions in the core measures section. Each question is unique, but may potentially require entry of patient record details, exemptions, and numerators/denominators if exclusion criteria are not met.
- After completing the core measures section, the EP will need to complete the menu set measures section. The first screen provides a comprehensive list of all measures and allows the EP to select menu measures for reporting, one of which must be from the public health section (even if an exclusion applies). The EP will then be asked to provide criteria for each menu measure that is selected.
- The next section contains the CQM questionnaires.

- Upon completion of all sections, the EP may proceed to the attestation summary page. Here the EP can review and change the core, menu, and CQMs that were entered in the questionnaire sections.
- Finally, the EP is required to agree to a series of statements related to the authenticity and accuracy of their attestation. Upon agreeing with all statements, the EP is directed to a confirmation page. After ensuring the information is correct, an attestation disclaimer is presented to the EP. Upon agreeing with this final disclaimer, the EP's attestation will be submitted and the system accepts or rejects the submission. Once accepted, the EP will qualify for an incentive payment for the reporting period and receive payment approximately four to eight weeks after successful submission.
- If the EP attestation is rejected, you may contact your Regional Extension Center (REC) for guidance.

How to use this guide

Below, we briefly discuss the structure of this book by highlighting key content and providing details about the layout of important information found throughout this guide.

"Final Rule" terminology

The ***Medicare and Medicaid Programs; Electronic Health Record Incentive Program—Stage 2 Final Rule*** (CMS Final Rule) and ***Health Information Technology: Standards, Implementation Specifications, and Certification Criteria for Electronic Health Record Technology, 2014 Edition; Revisions to the Permanent Certification Program for Health Information Technology Final Rule*** (ONC Final Rule) were released to the *Public Inspection Desk* on August 23, 2012 and published in the *Federal Register* on September 4, 2012.

In this guide, we refer to these rules as the ***CMS Stage 2 Final Rule*** and ***ONC 2014 Edition Standards & Certification Criteria Final Rule***. Also, there are instances where both of these rules are referred to as Stage 2 Final Rules, even though the ONC 2014 Edition Standards & Certification Criteria Final Rule is not explicitly tied to Stage 2, and, the CMS Stage 2 Final Rule includes program updates that impact Stage 1 Meaningful Use.

Callout boxes

Throughout this guide, you will find grey callout boxes denoted by one of the following: Note, Stage 2 Final Rule Impact, or Stay Up-to-Date.

- **Note** callouts provide topic and concept clarifications.
- **Stage 2 Final Rule Impact** callouts indicate important changes or updates to the program as a result of the Stage 2 Final Rules.
- **Stay Up-to-Date** callouts connect the reader to more information and provide online program updates.

Chapter 1: Stage 1 Core Set
Chapter 2: Stage 1 Menu Set

In the first two chapters of this guide, we outline relevant criteria for EPs during their first two years of participation in the program (Stage 1 Meaningful Use). The layout of these pages is consistent and we explain the content that appears on them in detail on the following pages.

Chapter 3: Clinical Quality Measures (CQMs)

In this chapter, we examine requirements that relate to Clinical Quality Measures and address program changes as a result of the Stage 2 Final Rules.

Chapter 4: Policies, Guidelines, and Audits

In this chapter, we help identify and define policies that will assist you with documenting your action plans and MU strategy as they relate to workload reductions. We also briefly touch upon considerations related to risks, audits, and record keeping.

Chapter 5: Criteria Level Exclusions

In this chapter, we examine a variety of exclusionary considerations by taking a look at specific Stage 1 criteria grouped by exclusion availability, provider activities, and attestation requirements.

Chapter 6: Stage 2 Final Rules

In this chapter, we review the Stage 2 Final Rules, examine the regulations, and take a look at the requirements set forth for Stage 2 Meaningful Use.

Chapter 7: Stage 2 Effects on Stage 1

In this chapter, we examine the impact of the Stage 2 Final Rules on Stage 1 Meaningful Use.

Chapter 8: Frequently Asked Questions

In this chapter, we address some of the most common questions about meaningful use as they relate to your first two years of the program—this compilation of questions and answers has been collected in part from the government program websites.

Chapter 9: Resources and Tools

In this chapter, we further prepare you for your first two years of meaningful use by taking a look at resources to help you along the way.

Sample Criteria Page Layout

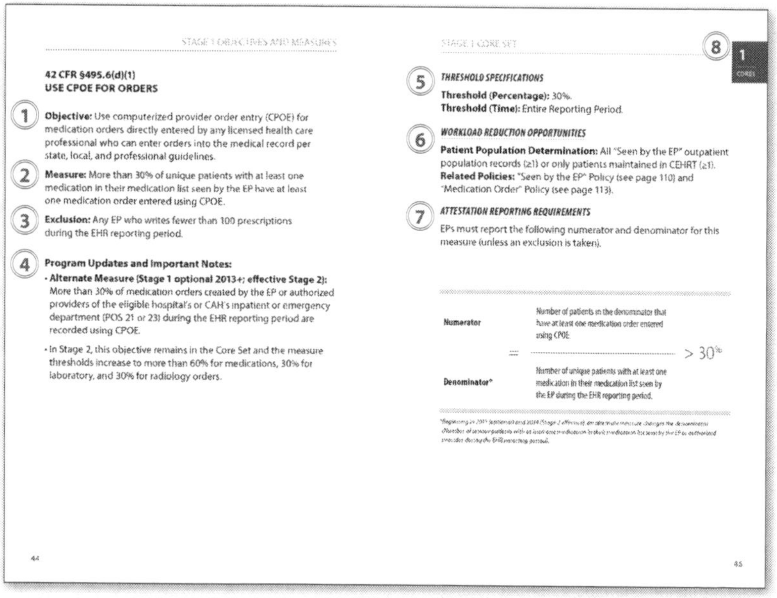

STAGE 1 OBJECTIVES AND MEASURES

42 CFR §495.6(d)(1)
USE CPOE FOR ORDERS

1 **Objective:** Use computerized provider order entry (CPOE) for medication orders directly entered by any licensed health care professional who can enter orders into the medical record per state, local, and professional guidelines.

2 **Measure:** More than 30% of unique patients with at least one medication in their medication list seen by the EP have at least one medication order entered using CPOE.

3 **Exclusion:** Any EP who writes fewer than 100 prescriptions during the EHR reporting period.

4 **Program Updates and Important Notes:**

- **Alternate Measure (Stage 1 optional 2013+; effective Stage 2):** More than 30% of medication orders created by the EP or authorized providers of the eligible hospital's or CAH's inpatient or emergency department (POS 21 or 23) during the EHR reporting period are recorded using CPOE.
- In Stage 2, this objective remains in the Core Set and the measure thresholds increase to more than 60% for medications, 30% for laboratory, and 30% for radiology orders.

44

STAGE 1 CORE SET

8 1 CORE

5 ***THRESHOLD SPECIFICATIONS***

Threshold (Percentage): 30%.
Threshold (Time): Entire Reporting Period.

6 ***WORKLOAD REDUCTION OPPORTUNITIES***

Patient Population Determination: All "Seen by the EP" outpatient population records (≥1) or only patients maintained in CEHRT (≥1).
Related Policies: "Seen by the EP" Policy (see page 110) and "Medication Order" Policy (see page 113).

7 ***ATTESTATION REPORTING REQUIREMENTS***

EPs must report the following numerator and denominator for this measure (unless an exclusion is taken).

Numerator	Number of patients in the denominator that have at least one medication order entered using CPOE.	
	=	> 30%
Denominator*	Number of unique patients with at least one medication in their medication list seen by the EP during the EHR reporting period.	

45

1. **Objective**
   Explains what EPs are required to achieve in order to be able to show they are meaningfully using their certified EHR.

2. **Measure**
   Details the minimum requirement EPs must meet, or surpass, in order to achieve each objective.

3. **Exclusion**
   Exempts an EP from having to meet a specific objective. If an EP meets the qualifications for exclusion, they will not have to report on that objective and can still receive an EHR incentive payment.

4. **Program Updates and Important Notes**
   Summarizes important updates and changes to Stage 1 criteria that were introduced with the release of the Stage 2 Final Rules. This section also contains notes and/or clarifications about the objective, measure, and/or exclusion.

5. **Threshold Specifications**
   Outlines minimum percentage of activity required in order to meet criteria and the associated time period.

6. **Workload Reduction Opportunities**
   Describes outpatient population determination and related group policies.

7. **Attestation Reporting Requirements**
   Provides attestation reporting requirements for each specific measure.

8. **Quick Reference Tab**
   Makes finding specific content easier and faster. A quick reference tab along the edge of every right-sided page marks each chapter in this guide. For Chapters 1 and 2, these tabs also contain a quick reference number so you can easily find individual Core and Menu Set criteria.

Part I:

STAGE 1 OBJECTIVES AND MEASURES

In Part I, we discuss the objectives and measures that make it possible to assess the effectiveness of the Medicare EHR Incentive Program. We take a look at the core set, menu set, and clinical quality measures that must be reported by EPs participating in the program and identify exclusion opportunities and policy guidance. We also review the Stage 2 Final Rules and the impact on Stage 1 criteria.

Part I:

STAGE 1 OBJECTIVES AND MEASURES

CHAPTER 1

Stage 1 Core Set

Read more about the core set objectives and measures.

To review core set objectives and measures online, obtain access to program updates, and review specifications related to EPs, scan the QR code above or go to **objectivesandmeasures.theMUguide.com**.

In this chapter, we examine core set requirements for Stage 1 Meaningful Use and take a detailed look at thresholds, data capture specifications, exclusionary considerations, and attestation reporting requirements for each measure. We also address changes to specific criteria, and associated implementation timeframes, as a result of the Stage 2 Final Rules.

Satisfying requirements of the Medicare EHR Incentive Program is determined by compliance with a variety of meaningful use measures. All EPs are required to report 15 core set measures except when exclusion criteria are met. The core set includes six measures eligible for exclusion.

Due to the one-size-fits-all approach of the government incentive programs, practices will need to adapt some of the core set requirements and acquire new data points to satisfy program requirements. Despite these core objectives and measures that do not perfectly align with all physician and specialist activities, exclusion opportunities do exist.

In addition to the incentive payments, your practice should seek other benefits of the program—better data structure, better practice management capabilities, and better information that can be preserved in your IT systems.

The Stage 1 Core Set includes 15 objectives and measures:

42 CFR §495.6(d)(1): USE CPOE FOR ORDERS*
42 CFR §495.6(d)(2): DRUG-DRUG, DRUG-ALLERGY INTERACTION CHECKS
42 CFR §495.6(d)(3): MAINTAIN AN UP-TO-DATE PROBLEM LIST
42 CFR §495.6(d)(4): E-PRESCRIBING*
42 CFR §495.6(d)(5): MAINTAIN ACTIVE MEDICATION LIST
42 CFR §495.6(d)(6): MAINTAIN ACTIVE MEDICATION ALLERGY LIST
42 CFR §495.6(d)(7): RECORD DEMOGRAPHICS
42 CFR §495.6(d)(8): RECORD AND CHART CHANGES IN VITAL SIGNS*
42 CFR §495.6(d)(9): RECORD SMOKING STATUS
42 CFR §495.6(d)(10): REPORT AMBULATORY CQMs*
42 CFR §495.6(d)(11): IMPLEMENT CLINICAL DECISION SUPPORT
42 CFR §495.6(d)(12): PROVIDE PATIENTS WITH AN ELECTRONIC COPY OF THEIR HEALTH INFORMATION*
42 CFR §495.6(d)(13): PROVIDE CLINICAL SUMMARIES
42 CFR §495.6(d)(14): CAPABILITY TO EXCHANGE KEY CLINICAL INFORMATION*
42 CFR §495.6(d)(15): PROTECT ELECTRONIC HEALTH INFORMATION

Stage 2 Final Rule Impact: Stage 2 Final Rules introduced a number changes or updates to some of the Stage 1 criteria. An asterisk (*) indicates a change notice for those specific Stage 1 criteria. Please refer to the core, menu, and CQM criteria in Chapters 1, 2 and 3 for specific details.

42 CFR §495.6(d)(1) USE CPOE FOR ORDERS

Objective: Use computerized provider order entry (CPOE) for medication orders directly entered by any licensed health care professional who can enter orders into the medical record per state, local, and professional guidelines.

Measure: More than 30% of unique patients with at least one medication in their medication list seen by the EP have at least one medication order entered using CPOE.

Exclusion: Any EP who writes fewer than 100 prescriptions during the EHR reporting period.

Program Updates and Important Notes:

- **Alternate Measure (Stage 1 optional 2013+; effective Stage 2):** More than 30% of medication orders created by the EP or authorized providers of the eligible hospital's or CAH's inpatient or emergency department (POS 21 or 23) during the EHR reporting period are recorded using CPOE.
- In Stage 2, this objective remains in the Core Set and the measure thresholds increase to more than 60% for medications, 30% for laboratory, and 30% for radiology orders.

THRESHOLD SPECIFICATIONS

Threshold (Percentage): 30%.
Threshold (Time): Entire Reporting Period.

WORKLOAD REDUCTION OPPORTUNITIES

Patient Population Determination: All "Seen by the EP" outpatient population records (≥1) or only patients maintained in CEHRT (≥1).
Related Policies: "Seen by the EP" Policy (see page 110) and "Medication Order" Policy (see page 113).

ATTESTATION REPORTING REQUIREMENTS

EPs must report the following numerator and denominator for this measure (unless an exclusion is taken).

Numerator	Number of patients in the denominator that have at least one medication order entered using CPOE.	
=	————————	> 30%
Denominator*	Number of unique patients with at least one medication in their medication list seen by the EP during the EHR reporting period.	

**Beginning in 2013 (optional) and 2014 (Stage 2 effective), an alternate measure changes the denominator (Number of unique patients with at least one medication in their medication list seen by the EP or authorized provider during the EHR reporting period).*

42 CFR §495.6(d)(2)
DRUG-DRUG, DRUG-ALLERGY INTERACTION CHECKS

Objective: Implement drug-drug and drug-allergy interaction checks.

Measure: The EP has enabled this functionality for the entire EHR reporting period.

Exclusion: None.

Program Updates and Important Notes:

- No Stage 1 changes introduced in Stage 2 Final Rules.
- In Stage 2, this objective remains in the Core Set and is incorporated into the **Implement Clinical Decision Support** objective.

THRESHOLD SPECIFICATIONS

Threshold (Percentage): Ongoing.
Threshold (Time): Entire Reporting Period.

WORKLOAD REDUCTION OPPORTUNITIES

Patient Population Determination: None; not a percentage-based measure.
Related Policies: None.

ATTESTATION REPORTING REQUIREMENTS

Yes/No Only. EPs must attest to having enabled drug-drug and drug-allergy interaction checks for the length of the reporting period to meet this measure (no exclusion available).

42 CFR §495.6(d)(3)
MAINTAIN AN UP-TO-DATE PROBLEM LIST

Objective: Maintain an up-to-date problem list of current and active diagnoses.

Measure: More than 80% of all unique patients seen by the EP have at least one entry or an indication that no problems are known for the patient recorded as structured data.

Exclusion: None.

Program Updates and Important Notes:

- No Stage 1 changes introduced in Stage 2 Final Rules.
- In Stage 2, this objective remains in the Core Set and is incorporated into the **Summary of Care for Transitions of Care or Referral** objective.

THRESHOLD SPECIFICATIONS

Threshold (Percentage): 80%.
Threshold (Time): Entire Reporting Period.

WORKLOAD REDUCTION OPPORTUNITIES

Patient Population Determination: All "Seen by the EP" outpatient population records (≥1).
Related Policies: "Seen by the EP" Policy (see page 110).

ATTESTATION REPORTING REQUIREMENTS

EPs must report the following numerator and denominator for this measure (no exclusion available).

Numerator	Number of patients in the denominator who have at least one entry or an indication that no problems are known for the patient recorded as structured data in their problem list.	
	=	> 80%
Denominator	Number of unique patients seen by the EP during the EHR reporting period.	

42 CFR §495.6(d)(4)
E-PRESCRIBING

Objective: Generate and transmit permissible prescriptions electronically (eRx).

Measure: More than 40% of all permissible prescriptions written by the EP are transmitted electronically using certified EHR technology.

Exclusion: Any EP who writes fewer than 100 prescriptions during the EHR reporting period.

Program Updates and Important Notes:

- **Additional Exclusion (Stage 1 effective 2013+):** Any EP who does not have a pharmacy within their organization and there are no pharmacies that accept electronic prescriptions within 10 miles of the EP's practice location at the start of his/her EHR reporting period.
- In Stage 2, this objective remains in the Core Set and the measure thresholds increase to more than 50% and must be compared to at least one drug formulary.

THRESHOLD SPECIFICATIONS

Threshold (Percentage): 40%.
Threshold (Time): Entire Reporting Period.

WORKLOAD REDUCTION OPPORTUNITIES

Patient Population Determination: All outpatient records or only patient populations maintained in CEHRT.
Related Policies: "Medication Order" Policy (see page 113).

ATTESTATION REPORTING REQUIREMENTS

EPs must report the following numerator and denominator for this measure (unless an exclusion is taken).

Numerator		Number of prescriptions in the denominator generated and transmitted electronically.	
	=	―――――	> 40%
Denominator		Number of prescriptions written for drugs requiring a prescription in order to be dispensed other than controlled substances during the EHR reporting period.	

42 CFR §495.6(d)(5)
MAINTAIN ACTIVE MEDICATION LIST

Objective: Maintain active medication list.

Measure: More than 80% of all unique patients seen by the EP have at least one entry (or an indication that the patient is not currently prescribed any medication) recorded as structured data.

Exclusion: None.

Program Updates and Important Notes:

- No Stage 1 changes introduced in Stage 2 Final Rules.
- In Stage 2, this objective remains in the Core Set and is incorporated into the **Summary of Care for Transitions of Care or Referral** objective.

THRESHOLD SPECIFICATIONS

Threshold (Percentage): 80%.
Threshold (Time): Entire Reporting Period.

WORKLOAD REDUCTION OPPORTUNITIES

Patient Population Determination: All "Seen by the EP" outpatient population records (≥1).
Related Policies: "Seen by the EP" Policy (see page 110).

ATTESTATION REPORTING REQUIREMENTS

EPs must report the following numerator and denominator for this measure (no exclusion available).

Numerator	Number of patients in the denominator who have a medication (or an indication that the patient is not currently prescribed any medication) recorded as structured data.	
=	———	> 80%
Denominator	Number of unique patients seen by the EP during the EHR reporting period.	

42 CFR §495.6(d)(6)
MAINTAIN ACTIVE MEDICATION ALLERGY LIST

Objective: Maintain active medication allergy list.

Measure: More than 80% of all unique patients seen by the EP have at least one entry (or an indication that the patient has no known medication allergies) recorded as structured data.

Exclusion: None.

Program Updates and Important Notes:

- No Stage 1 changes introduced in Stage 2 Final Rules.
- In Stage 2, this objective remains in the Core Set and is incorporated into the **Summary of Care for Transitions of Care or Referral** objective.

THRESHOLD SPECIFICATIONS

Threshold (Percentage): 80%.
Threshold (Time): Entire Reporting Period.

WORKLOAD REDUCTION OPPORTUNITIES

Patient Population Determination: All "Seen by the EP" outpatient population records (≥1).
Related Policies: "Seen by the EP" Policy (see page 110).

ATTESTATION REPORTING REQUIREMENTS

EPs must report the following numerator and denominator for this measure (no exclusion available).

Numerator	Number of unique patients in the denominator who have at least one entry (or an indication that the patient has no known medication allergies) recorded as structured data in their medication allergy list.	
	=	> 80%
Denominator	Number of unique patients seen by the EP during the EHR reporting period.	

42 CFR §495.6(d)(7)
RECORD DEMOGRAPHICS

Objective: Record demographics: preferred language, gender, race, ethnicity, date of birth.

Measure: More than 50% of all unique patients seen by the EP have demographics recorded as structured data.

Exclusion: None.

Program Updates and Important Notes:

- No Stage 1 changes introduced in Stage 2 Final Rules.
- In Stage 2, this objective remains in the Core Set and the measure thresholds increase to more than 80%.

THRESHOLD SPECIFICATIONS

Threshold (Percentage): 50%.
Threshold (Time): Entire Reporting Period.

WORKLOAD REDUCTION OPPORTUNITIES

Patient Population Determination: All "Seen by the EP" outpatient population records (≥1).
Related Policies: "Seen by the EP" Policy (see page 110).

ATTESTATION REPORTING REQUIREMENTS

EPs must report the following numerator and denominator for this measure (no exclusion available).

Numerator	Number of patients in the denominator who have all the elements of demographics (or a specific exclusion if the patient declined to provide one or more elements or if recording an element is contrary to state law) recorded as structured data.	
=	─────────	> 50%
Denominator	Number of unique patients seen by the EP during the EHR reporting period.	

42 CFR §495.6(d)(8)
RECORD AND CHART CHANGES IN VITAL SIGNS

Objective: Record and chart changes in vital signs: height, weight, blood pressure. Calculate and display BMI, plot and display growth charts for children 2–20 years (including BMI).

Measure: More than 50% of all unique patients age 2 and over seen by the EP have height, weight, and blood pressure recorded as structured data.

Exclusion: Any EP who either sees no patients 2 years or older, or who believes that all three vital signs of height, weight, and blood pressure of their patients have no relevance in their scope of practice.

Program Updates and Important Notes:

- **Alternate Measure (Stage 1 optional 2013; effective 2014+):** More than 50% of all unique patients seen by the EP or admitted to the eligible hospital's or CAH's inpatient or emergency department (POS 21 or 23) during the EHR reporting period have blood pressure (for patients age 3 and over only) and height and weight (for all ages) recorded as structured data.
- **Alternate Exclusion (Stage 1 optional 2013; effective 2014+):** Any EP who (1) sees no patients 3 years or older is excluded from recording blood pressure; (2) believes that all three vital signs of height, weight, and blood pressure have no relevance to their scope of practice is excluded from recording them; (3) believes that height and weight are relevant to their scope of practice, but blood pressure is not, is excluded from recording blood pressure; or (4) believes that blood pressure is relevant to their scope of practice, but height and weight are not, is excluded from recording height and weight.
- In Stage 2, this objective remains in the Core Set and the measure thresholds increase to more than 80%.

THRESHOLD SPECIFICATIONS

Threshold (Percentage): 50%.
Threshold (Time): Entire Reporting Period.

WORKLOAD REDUCTION OPPORTUNITIES

Patient Population Determination: All "Seen by the EP" outpatient population records (≥1) or only patients maintained in CEHRT (≥1).
Related Policies: "Seen by the EP" Policy (see page 110) and "Vital Sign" Policy (see page 112).

ATTESTATION REPORTING REQUIREMENTS

EPs must report the following numerator and denominator for this measure (unless an exclusion is taken).

Numerator*	=	Number of patients in the denominator who have at least one entry of their height, weight and blood pressure are recorded as structured data.	> 50%
Denominator*		Number of unique patients age 2 or over seen by the EP during the EHR reporting period.	

**Beginning in 2013 (optional) and 2014+ (effective), an alternate measure changes the numerator (Number of patients in the denominator who have at least one entry of their height/length and weight (all ages) and/or blood pressure (ages 3 and over) recorded as structured data) and denominator (Number of unique patients seen by the EP or admitted to an eligible hospital's or CAH's inpatient or emergency department (POS 21 or 23) during the EHR reporting period) for attestation.*

42 CFR §495.6(d)(9)
RECORD SMOKING STATUS

Objective: Record smoking status for patients 13 years old or older.

Measure: More than 50% of all unique patients 13 years old or older seen by the EP have smoking status recorded as structured data.

Exclusion: Any EP who sees no patients 13 years and older.

Program Updates and Important Notes:

- No Stage 1 changes introduced in Stage 2 Final Rules.
- In Stage 2, this objective remains in the Core Set and the measure thresholds increase to more than 80%.

THRESHOLD SPECIFICATIONS

Threshold (Percentage): 50%.
Threshold (Time): Entire Reporting Period.

WORKLOAD REDUCTION OPPORTUNITIES

Patient Population Determination: All "Seen by the EP" outpatient population records (≥1) or only patients maintained in CEHRT (≥1).
Related Policies: "Seen by the EP" Policy (see page 110).

ATTESTATION REPORTING REQUIREMENTS

EPs must report the following numerator and denominator for this measure (unless an exclusion is taken).

Numerator		Number of patients in the denominator with smoking status recorded as structured data.
	=	——————— > 50%
Denominator		Number of unique patients age 13 or older seen by the EP during the EHR reporting period.

42 CFR §495.6(d)(10)
REPORT AMBULATORY CQMs

Objective: Report ambulatory clinical quality measures to CMS or the States.

Measure: For 2011, provide aggregate numerator and denominator, and exclusions through attestation as required by CMS and for 2012, electronically submit the CQMs as required by CMS.

Exclusion: None.

Program Updates and Important Notes:

- **Eliminated/Absorbed into MU Definition (Stage 1 effective 2013+):** Due to provisions in the CMS Stage 2 Final Rule, 42 CFR §495.6(d)(10) will no longer be a separate standalone objective beginning in 2013. 42 CFR §495.6(d)(10) has been incorporated directly into the definition of meaningful use, and as such, program participants are still required to report CQMs in order to achieve meaningful use.
- In Stage 2, this objective is no longer separate, but providers must still submit CQMs to CMS in order to achieve meaningful use.

THRESHOLD SPECIFICATIONS

Threshold (Percentage): None.
Threshold (Time): Entire Reporting Period.

WORKLOAD REDUCTION OPPORTUNITIES

Patient Population Determination: All outpatient records or only patient populations maintained in CEHRT.
Related Policies: "CQM Selection" Policy (see page 114).

ATTESTATION REPORTING REQUIREMENTS

Yes/No Only. EPs must attest to reporting to CMS ambulatory clinical quality measures selected by CMS in the manner specified by CMS to meet the measure (no exclusion available).

42 CFR §495.6(d)(11)
IMPLEMENT CLINICAL DECISION SUPPORT

Objective: Implement one clinical decision support rule relevant to specialty or high clinical priority along with the ability to track compliance with that rule.

Measure: Implement one clinical decision support rule.

Exclusion: None.

Program Updates and Important Notes:

- No Stage 1 changes introduced in Stage 2 Final Rules.
- In Stage 2, this objective remains in the Core Set and is combined with drug-drug and drug-allergy interaction checks and the measure thresholds increase to 5 clinical decision support interventions.

THRESHOLD SPECIFICATIONS

Threshold (Percentage): Ongoing.
Threshold (Time): Entire Reporting Period.

WORKLOAD REDUCTION OPPORTUNITIES

Patient Population Determination: None; not a percentage-based measure.
Related Policies: "Clinical Decision Support" Policy (see page 114).

ATTESTATION REPORTING REQUIREMENTS

Yes/No Only. EPs must attest to having implemented one clinical decision support rule for the length of the reporting period to meet the measure (no exclusion available).

42 CFR §495.6(d)(12)
PROVIDE PATIENTS WITH AN ELECTRONIC COPY OF THEIR HEALTH INFORMATION

Objective: Provide patients with an electronic copy of their health information (including diagnostic test results, problem list, medication lists, medication allergies) upon request.

Measure: More than 50% of all patients who request an electronic copy of their health information are provided it within three business days.

Exclusion: Any EP that has no requests from patients or their agents for an electronic copy of patient health information during the EHR reporting period.

Program Updates and Important Notes:

- Starting in 2014, 42 CFR §495.6(d)(12) will be replaced with a new objective and measure that better aligns with 2014 CEHRT capabilities.
  - **New Objective (replaces current criteria; Stage 1 effective 2014+):** Provide patients the ability to view online, download and transmit their health information within 4 business days of the information being available to the EP.
  - **New Measure (replaces current criteria; Stage 1 effective 2014+):** More than 50% of all unique patients seen by the EP during the EHR reporting period are provided timely (within 4 business days after the information is available to the EP) online access to their health information subject to the EP's discretion to withhold certain information.
- In Stage 2, this new objective remains in the Core Set as the **Patient Access to Online Health Information** objective and requires that more than 5% of patients access their information.

THRESHOLD SPECIFICATIONS

Threshold (Percentage): 50%.
Threshold (Time): 3 Business Days (4 Business Days in 2014+).

WORKLOAD REDUCTION OPPORTUNITIES

Patient Population Determination: All outpatient records or only patient populations maintained in CEHRT.
Related Policies: "Seen by the EP" Policy (effective 2014+; see page 110), "Patient Request" Policy (see page 115), and "Physician Discretion" Policy (see page 117).

ATTESTATION REPORTING REQUIREMENTS

EPs must report the following numerator and denominator for this measure (unless an exclusion is taken).

Numerator*	=	Number of patients in the denominator who receive an electronic copy of their electronic health information within three business days.	> 50%
Denominator*		Number of patients of the EP who request an electronic copy of their electronic health information four business days prior to the end of the EHR reporting period.	

**Beginning in 2014+, 42 CFR §495.6(d)(12) will be replaced with a new objective and measure that better aligns with 2014 CEHRT capabilities. As a result, a new numerator (The number of patients in the denominator who have timely (within 4 business days after the information is available to the EP) online access to their health information) and denominator (Number of unique patients seen by the EP during the EHR reporting period) have been introduced.*

42 CFR §495.6(d)(13)
PROVIDE CLINICAL SUMMARIES

Objective: Provide clinical summaries for patients for each office visit.

Measure: Clinical summaries provided to patients for more than 50% of all office visits within three business days.

Exclusion: Any EP who has no office visits during the EHR reporting period.

Program Updates and Important Notes:

- No Stage 1 changes introduced in Stage 2 Final Rules.
- In Stage 2, this objective remains in the Core Set and the measure thresholds remain at more than 50%, but must be provided within 1 business day.

THRESHOLD SPECIFICATIONS

Threshold (Percentage): 50%.
Threshold (Time): 3 Business Days.

WORKLOAD REDUCTION OPPORTUNITIES

Patient Population Determination: All "Office Visit" outpatient population records (≥0) or only patients maintained in CEHRT (≥0).
Related Policies: "Office Visit" Policy (see page 112).

ATTESTATION REPORTING REQUIREMENTS

EPs must report the following numerator and denominator for this measure (unless an exclusion is taken).

Numerator	Number of office visits in the denominator for which the patient is provided a clinical summary within three business days.	
=	———	> 50%
Denominator	Number of office visits by the EP during the EHR reporting period.	

42 CFR §495.6(d)(14)
CAPABILITY TO EXCHANGE KEY CLINICAL INFORMATION

Objective: Capability to exchange key clinical information (for example: problem list, medication list, medication allergies, diagnostic test results) among providers of care and patient authorized entities electronically.

Measure: Performed at least one test of certified EHR technology's capacity to electronically exchange key clinical information.

Exclusion: None.

Program Updates and Important Notes:

- **Eliminated (Stage 1 effective 2013+):** Effective 2013, this Stage 1 requirement has been removed in favor of the more robust, actual use case of electronic exchange through a summary of care record following each transition of care or referral.
- In Stage 2, this objective no longer exists as it has been eliminated from Stage 1 effective 2013.

THRESHOLD SPECIFICATIONS

Threshold (Percentage): Once.
Threshold (Time): During Reporting Period.

WORKLOAD REDUCTION OPPORTUNITIES

Patient Population Determination: None; not a percentage-based measure.
Related Policies: "Information Exchange Methodology" Policy (see page 115).

ATTESTATION REPORTING REQUIREMENTS

Yes/No Only. EPs must attest to having performed at least one test of certified EHR technology's capacity to electronically exchange key clinical information during the EHR reporting period to meet this measure (no exclusion available).

42 CFR §495.6(d)(15)
PROTECT ELECTRONIC HEALTH INFORMATION

Objective: Protect electronic health information created or maintained by the certified EHR technology through the implementation of appropriate technical capabilities.

Measure: Conduct or review a security risk analysis per 45 CFR §164.308(a)(1) and implement security updates as necessary and correct identified security deficiencies as part of its risk management process.

Exclusion: None.

Program Updates and Important Notes:

- No Stage 1 changes introduced in Stage 2 Final Rules.
- In Stage 2, this objective remains in the Core Set.

THRESHOLD SPECIFICATIONS

Threshold (Percentage): Once.
Threshold (Time): During Reporting Period.

WORKLOAD REDUCTION OPPORTUNITIES

Patient Population Determination: None; not a percentage-based measure.
Related Policies: "Security Risk Analysis Methodology" Policy (see page 116).

ATTESTATION REPORTING REQUIREMENTS

Yes/No Only. EPs must attest to having conducted or reviewed a security risk analysis in accordance with the requirements under 45 CFR §164.308(a)(1) and implemented security updates as necessary and corrected identified security deficiencies prior to or during the EHR reporting period to meet this measure (no exclusion available).

Part I:

STAGE 1 OBJECTIVES AND MEASURES

CHAPTER 2

Stage 1 Menu Set

Read more about the menu set objectives and measures.

To review menu set objectives and measures online, obtain access to program updates, and review specifications related to EPs, scan the QR code above or go to **objectivesandmeasures.theMUguide.com**.

In this chapter, we examine menu set requirements for Stage 1 Meaningful Use and take a detailed look at thresholds, data capture specifications, exclusionary considerations, and attestation reporting requirements for each measure. We also address changes to specific criteria, and associated implementation timeframes, as a result of the Stage 2 Final Rules.

Satisfying the requirements of the Medicare EHR Incentive Program is determined by compliance with a variety of additional measures beyond the core set. All EPs are required to report five out of 10 menu set measures except when exclusion criteria are met. If an EP meets the exclusion criteria for one menu set measure, they would select four of the remaining nine measures; if an EP meets exclusion criteria for two menu set measures, they would select three of the remaining eight; if an EP meets exclusion criteria for three menu set measures, they would select two of the remaining seven; and so on.

Stage 2 Final Rule Impact: Beginning in 2014, EPs will no longer be permitted to count an exclusion toward the minimum of 5 menu objectives in which they must report if there are other menu objectives for which they can select. Refer to Chapter 6 for more information about new Stage 2 Menu Set criteria and Chapter 7 for changes to Stage 1 criteria.

As with the core set, you may need to adapt some of the menu set requirements and acquire new data points to satisfy program requirements. The menu set offers a greater opportunity for exclusions and more flexibility than the core set.

The Stage 1 Menu Set includes 10 objectives and measures:

42 CFR §495.6(e)(1): IMPLEMENT DRUG-FORMULARY CHECKS
42 CFR §495.6(e)(2): INCORPORATE CLINICAL LAB TEST RESULTS
42 CFR §495.6(e)(3): GENERATE LISTS OF PATIENTS WITH SPECIFIC CONDITIONS
42 CFR §495.6(e)(4): SEND REMINDERS TO PATIENTS
42 CFR §495.6(e)(5): PROVIDE TIMELY ACCESS TO PATIENT HEALTH INFORMATION*
42 CFR §495.6(e)(6): PATIENT-SPECIFIC EDUCATION RESOURCES
42 CFR §495.6(e)(7): MEDICATION RECONCILIATION
42 CFR §495.6(e)(8): PROVIDE SUMMARY OF CARE RECORD FOR TRANSITIONS OF CARE OR REFERRAL
42 CFR §495.6(e)(9): CAPBILITY TO SUBMIT ELECTRONIC DATA TO IMMUNIZATION REGISTRIES*
42 CFR §495.6(e)(10): CAPABILITY TO SUBMIT ELECTRONIC SYNDROMIC SURVEILLANCE DATA*

Stage 2 Final Rule Impact: Stage 2 Final Rules introduced a number changes or updates to some of the Stage 1 criteria. An asterisk (*) indicates a change notice for those specific Stage 1 criteria. Please refer to the core, menu, and CQM criteria in Chapters 1, 2 and 3 for specific details.

42 CFR §495.6(e)(1)
IMPLEMENT DRUG-FORMULARY CHECKS

Objective: Implement drug-formulary checks.

Measure: The EP has enabled this functionality and has access to at least one internal or external formulary for the entire EHR reporting period.

Exclusion: Any EP who writes fewer than 100 prescriptions during the EHR reporting period.

Program Updates and Important Notes:

- No Stage 1 changes introduced in Stage 2 Final Rules.
- In Stage 2, this moves from the Menu Set to the Core Set and is incorporated into the **e-Prescribing** objective.

THRESHOLD SPECIFICATIONS

Threshold (Percentage): Ongoing.
Threshold (Time): Entire Reporting Period.

WORKLOAD REDUCTION OPPORTUNITIES

Patient Population Determination: None; not a percentage-based measure.
Related Policies: "Medication Order" Policy (see page 113).

ATTESTATION REPORTING REQUIREMENTS

Yes/No Only. EPs must attest to having enabled this functionality and having had access to at least one internal or external formulary for the entire EHR reporting period to meet this measure (EPs claiming an exclusion must enter '0' in the "Exclusion" box to attest to exclusion from this requirement).

42 CFR §495.6(e)(2)
INCORPORATE CLINICAL LAB TEST RESULTS

Objective: Incorporate clinical lab test results into certified EHR technology as structured data.

Measure: More than 40% of all clinical lab test results ordered by the EP during the EHR reporting period whose results are either in a positive/negative or numerical format are incorporated in certified EHR technology as structured data.

Exclusion: An EP who orders no lab tests whose results are either in a positive/negative or numeric format during the EHR reporting period.

Program Updates and Important Notes:

- No Stage 1 changes introduced in Stage 2 Final Rules.
- In Stage 2, this objective moves from the Menu Set to the Core Set and the measure thresholds increase to more than 55%.

THRESHOLD SPECIFICATIONS

Threshold (Percentage): 40%.
Threshold (Time): Entire Reporting Period.

WORKLOAD REDUCTION OPPORTUNITIES

Patient Population Determination: All outpatient records or only patient populations maintained in CEHRT.
Related Policies: "Lab Order" Policy (see page 113).

ATTESTATION REPORTING REQUIREMENTS

EPs must report the following numerator and denominator for this measure (unless an exclusion is taken).

Numerator		Number of lab test results whose results are expressed in a positive or negative affirmation or as a number which are incorporated as structured data.	
	=	————————	> 40%
Denominator		Number of lab tests ordered during the EHR reporting period by the EP whose results are expressed in a positive or negative affirmation or as a number.	

42 CFR §495.6(e)(3)
GENERATE LISTS OF PATIENTS WITH SPECIFIC CONDITIONS

Objective: Generate lists of patients by specific conditions to use for quality improvement, reduction of disparities, research, or outreach.

Measure: Generate at least one report listing patients of the EP with a specific condition.

Exclusion: None.

Program Updates and Important Notes:

- No Stage 1 changes introduced in Stage 2 Final Rules.
- In Stage 2, this objective moves from the Menu Set to the Core Set.

THRESHOLD SPECIFICATIONS

Threshold (Percentage): Once.
Threshold (Time): During Reporting Period.

WORKLOAD REDUCTION OPPORTUNITIES

Patient Population Determination: All outpatient records or only patient populations maintained in CEHRT.
Related Policies: "Patient List" Policy (see page 116).

ATTESTATION REPORTING REQUIREMENTS

Yes/No Only. EPs must attest YES to having generated at least one report listing patients of the EP with a specific condition to meet this measure (no exclusion available).

42 CFR §495.6(e)(4)
SEND REMINDERS TO PATIENTS

Objective: Send reminders to patients per patient preference for preventive/follow-up care.

Measure: More than 20% of all unique patients 65 years or older or 5 years old or younger were sent an appropriate reminder during the EHR reporting period.

Exclusion: An EP who has no patients 65 years or older or 5 years old or younger with records maintained using certified EHR technology.

Program Updates and Important Notes:

- No Stage 1 changes introduced in Stage 2 Final Rules.
- In Stage 2, this objective moves from the Menu Set to the Core Set as the **Preventative Reminders** objective and requires EPs to provide reminders for preventative/follow-up care for more than 10% of patients with two or more office visits in the last two years.

THRESHOLD SPECIFICATIONS

Threshold (Percentage): 20%.
Threshold (Time): Entire Reporting Period.

WORKLOAD REDUCTION OPPORTUNITIES

Patient Population Determination: All outpatient records or only patient populations maintained in CEHRT.
Related Policies: "Patient Age" Policy (see page 117).

ATTESTATION REPORTING REQUIREMENTS

EPs must report the following numerator and denominator for this measure (unless an exclusion is taken).

Numerator	Number of patients in the denominator who were sent the appropriate reminder.	
	= ————————	> 20%
Denominator	Number of unique patients 65 years old or older or 5 years older or younger.	

42 CFR §495.6(e)(5)
PROVIDE TIMELY ACCESS TO PATIENT HEALTH INFORMATION

Objective: Provide patients with timely electronic access to their health information (including lab results, problem list, medication lists, medication allergies) within four business days of the information being available to the EP.

Measure: More than 10% of all unique patients seen by the EP are provided timely (available to the patient within four business days of being updated in the certified EHR technology) electronic access to their health information subject to the EP's discretion to withhold certain information.

Exclusion: Any EP that neither orders nor creates any of the information listed at 45 CFR §170.304(g)—enable a user to provide patients with online access to their clinical information, including, at a minimum, lab test results, problem list, medication list, and medication allergy list—during the EHR reporting period.

Program Updates and Important Notes:

- Starting in 2014, 42 CFR §495.6(e)(5) will be replaced with a new objective and measure that better aligns with 2014 CEHRT capabilities.
  - **New Objective (replaces current criteria; moves to Core Set; Stage 1 effective 2014+):** Provide patients the ability to view online, download and transmit their health information within 4 business days of the information being available to the EP.
  - **New Measure (replaces current criteria; moves to Core Set; Stage 1 effective 2014+):** More than 50% of all unique patients seen by the EP during the EHR reporting period are provided timely (within 4 business days after the information is available to the EP) online access to their health information subject to the EP's discretion to withhold certain information.
- In Stage 2, this new objective resides in the Core Set as the **Patient Access to Online Health Information** objective.

THRESHOLD SPECIFICATIONS

Threshold (Percentage): 10% (50% in 2014+).
Threshold (Time): 4 Business Days.

WORKLOAD REDUCTION OPPORTUNITIES

Patient Population Determination: All "Seen by the EP" outpatient population records (≥1).
Related Policies: "Seen by the EP" Policy (see page 110) and "Physician Discretion" Policy (see page 117).

ATTESTATION REPORTING REQUIREMENTS

EPs must report the following numerator and denominator for this measure (unless an exclusion is taken).

Numerator*	=	Number of patients in the denominator who have timely (available to the patient within four business days of being updated in the certified EHR technology) electronic access to their health information online.	> 10%*
Denominator*		Number of unique patients seen by the EP during the EHR reporting period.	

**Beginning in 2014+, 42 CFR §495.6(e)(5) will be replaced with a new objective and measure that better aligns with 2014 CEHRT capabilities. As a result, a new numerator (The number of patients in the denominator who have timely (within 4 business days after the information is available to the EP) online access to their health information) and denominator (Number of unique patients seen by the EP during the EHR reporting period) have been introduced. Also, the threshold percentage increases from 10% to 50%.*

42 CFR §495.6(e)(6)
PATIENT-SPECIFIC EDUCATION RESOURCES

Objective: Use certified EHR technology to identify patient-specific education resources and provide those resources to the patient if appropriate.

Measure: More than 10% of all unique patients seen by the EP during the EHR reporting period are provided patient-specific education resources.

Exclusion: None.

Program Updates and Important Notes:

- No Stage 1 changes introduced in Stage 2 Final Rules.
- In Stage 2, this objective moves from the Menu Set to the Core Set.

THRESHOLD SPECIFICATIONS

Threshold (Percentage): 10%.
Threshold (Time): Entire Reporting Period.

WORKLOAD REDUCTION OPPORTUNITIES

Patient Population Determination: All "Seen by the EP" outpatient population records (≥1).
Related Policies: "Seen by the EP" Policy (see page 110).

ATTESTATION REPORTING REQUIREMENTS

EPs must report the following numerator and denominator for this measure (no exclusion available).

Numerator	Number of patients in the denominator who are provided patient-specific education resources.	
	= ――――――――――	> 10%
Denominator	Number of unique patients seen by the EP during the EHR reporting period.	

42 CFR §495.6(e)(7)
MEDICATION RECONCILIATION

Objective: The EP who receives a patient from another setting of care or provider of care or believes an encounter is relevant should perform medication reconciliation.

Measure: The EP performs medication reconciliation for more than 50% of transitions of care in which the patient is transitioned into the care of the EP.

Exclusion: An EP who was not the recipient of any transitions of care during the reporting period.

Program Updates and Important Notes:

- No Stage 1 changes introduced in Stage 2 Final Rules.
- In Stage 2, this objective moves from the Menu Set to the Core Set.

THRESHOLD SPECIFICATIONS

Threshold (Percentage): 50%.
Threshold (Time): Entire Reporting Period.

WORKLOAD REDUCTION OPPORTUNITIES

Patient Population Determination: All outpatient records or only patient populations maintained in CEHRT.
Related Policies: "Transitions of Care" Policy (see page 117).

ATTESTATION REPORTING REQUIREMENTS

EPs must report the following numerator and denominator for this measure (unless an exclusion is taken).

Numerator		Number of transitions of care in the denominator where medication reconciliation was performed.	
	=	————	> 50%
Denominator		Number of transitions of care during the EHR reporting period for which the EP was the receiving party of the transition.	

42 CFR §495.6(e)(8)
PROVIDE SUMMARY OF CARE RECORD FOR TRANSITIONS OF CARE OR REFERRAL

Objective: The EP who transitions their patient to another setting of care or refers their patient to another provider of care should provide summary of care record for each transition of care or referral.

Measure: The EP who transitions their patient to another setting of care or provider of care provides a summary of care record for more than 50% of transitions of care and referrals.

Exclusion: An EP who neither transfers a patient to another setting nor refers a patient to another provider during the EHR reporting period.

Program Updates and Important Notes:

- No Stage 1 changes introduced in Stage 2 Final Rules.
- In Stage 2, this objective moves from the Menu Set to the Core Set as the **Summary of Care for Transitions of Care or Referral** objective.

THRESHOLD SPECIFICATIONS

Threshold (Percentage): 50%.
Threshold (Time): Entire Reporting Period.

WORKLOAD REDUCTION OPPORTUNITIES

Patient Population Determination: All outpatient records or only patient populations maintained in CEHRT.
Related Policies: "Transitions of Care" Policy (see page 117).

ATTESTATION REPORTING REQUIREMENTS

EPs must report the following numerator and denominator for this measure (unless an exclusion is taken).

Numerator		Number of transitions of care and referrals in the denominator where a summary of care record was provided.	
	=	————————	> 50%
Denominator		Number of transitions of care and referrals during the EHR reporting period for which the EP was the transferring or referring provider.	

42 CFR §495.6(e)(9)
CAPBILITY TO SUBMIT ELECTRONIC DATA TO IMMUNIZATION REGISTRIES

Objective: Capability to submit electronic data to immunization registries or Immunization Information Systems and actual submission in accordance with applicable law and practice.

Measure: Performed at least one test of certified EHR technology's capacity to submit electronic data to immunization registries and follow up submission if the test is successful (unless none of the immunization registries to which the EP submits such information have the capacity to receive the information electronically).

Exclusion: An EP who administers no immunizations during the EHR reporting period or where no immunization registry has the capacity to receive the information electronically.

Program Updates and Important Notes:

- **New Objective (replaces current criteria; Stage 1 effective 2013+):** Capability to submit electronic data to immunization registries or Immunization Information Systems and actual submission in accordance with applicable law and practice, except where prohibited by law.
- In Stage 2, this objective moves from the Menu Set to the Core Set and requires successful ongoing transmission of immunization data for the entire EHR reporting period.

THRESHOLD SPECIFICATIONS

Threshold (Percentage): Once.
Threshold (Time): During Reporting Period.

WORKLOAD REDUCTION OPPORTUNITIES

Patient Population Determination: None; not a percentage-based measure.
Related Policies: "Immunization Administration" Policy (see page 118).

ATTESTATION REPORTING REQUIREMENTS

Yes/No Only. EPs must attest to having performed at least one test of certified EHR technology's capacity to submit electronic data to immunization registries and follow up submission if the test was successful (unless none of the immunization registries to which the EP submits such information has the capacity to receive the information electronically) to meet this measure (unless an exclusion is taken).

42 CFR §495.6(e)(10) CAPABILITY TO SUBMIT ELECTRONIC SYNDROMIC SURVEILLANCE DATA

Objective: Capability to submit electronic syndromic surveillance data to public health agencies and actual submission in accordance with applicable law and practice.

Measure: Performed at least one test of certified EHR technology's capacity to provide electronic syndromic surveillance data to public health agencies and follow-up submission if the test is successful (unless none of the public health agencies to which an EP submits such information have the capacity to receive the information electronically).

Exclusion: An EP who does not collect any reportable syndromic information on their patients during the EHR reporting period or does not submit such information to any public health agency that has the capacity to receive the information electronically.

Program Updates and Important Notes:

- **New Objective (replaces current criteria; Stage 1 effective 2013+):** Capability to submit electronic syndromic surveillance data to public health agencies and actual submission in accordance with applicable law and practice, except where prohibited.
- In Stage 2, this objective remains in the Menu Set and requires successful ongoing transmission of syndromic surveillance data for the entire EHR reporting period.

THRESHOLD SPECIFICATIONS

Threshold (Percentage): Once.
Threshold (Time): During Reporting Period.

WORKLOAD REDUCTION OPPORTUNITIES

Patient Population Determination: None; not a percentage-based measure.
Related Policies: "Syndromic Surveillance" Policy (see page 118).

ATTESTATION REPORTING REQUIREMENTS

Yes/No Only. EPs must attest to having performed at least one test of certified EHR technology's capacity to submit electronic syndromic surveillance data to public health agencies and follow up submission if the test was successful (unless none of the public health agencies to which the EP submits such information has the capacity to receive the information electronically) to meet this measure (unless an exclusion is taken).

Part I:

STAGE 1 OBJECTIVES AND MEASURES

CHAPTER 3

Clinical Quality Measures (CQMs)

Read more about the clinical quality measures (CQMs).

To review clinical quality measures (CQMs) online, obtain access to program updates, and review specifications related to EPs, scan the QR code above or go to **cqms.theMUguide.com**.

In this chapter, we examine requirements that relate to Clinical Quality Measures and address program changes as a result of the Stage 2 Final Rules.

Under provisions of the CMS Stage 1 Final Rule, core objective 42 CFR §495.6(d)(10) requires providers to report clinical quality measures to CMS. With the CMS Stage 2 Final Rule, this core objective was removed and CQMs have been incorporated into the definition of a meaningful user. As such, EPs are still required to report CQM data in order to achieve meaningful use. And, starting in 2014, all providers must meet CY2014 CQM criteria regardless of the MU stage in which they are participating.

Prior to 2014: Clinical Quality Measures (CQMs)

To meet program requirements and successfully demonstrate meaningful use prior to 2014, EPs are required to report clinical quality measures in addition to the core set and menu set measures. In these years, EPs only have to demonstrate a total of six of the 44 clinical quality measures: three core/alternate core measures and three discretionary measures from the remaining 38 measures.

There are percentage-based measures that require the collection of numerator and denominator information to calculate and determine if minimum thresholds are met. If an EP has a denominator of zero for all core and alternate core measures, they could comply by reporting zeros. It is important to note that EPs must report this information even if they have no patients in the denominator.

Note: Stage 1 CQM reporting will remain the same through 2013 and the new CQM reporting model will go into effect beginning in 2014 for all program participants.

The following is a list of the 44 CQMs for reporting prior to 2014.

CQM CORE/ALTERNATE SET (6) CARDIAC, TOBACCO, OBESITY, IMMUNIZATION

- CORE: Hypertension Blood Pressure Measurement (NQF 0013)
- CORE: Tobacco Use Assessment and Cessation Intervention (NQF 0028)
- CORE: Adult Weight Screening and Follow-up (NQF 0421, PQRI 128)
- ALTERNATE: Weight Assessment and Counseling for Children and Adolescents (NQF 0024)
- ALTERNATE: Influenza Immunization for Patients 50 or Older (NQF 0041, PQRI 110)
- ALTERNATE: Childhood Immunization Status (NQF 0038)

CQM MENU SET (10 OF 38) CARDIAC

- Heart Failure: ACE Inhibitor Therapy
- Heart Failure: Warfarin Therapy Patients with Atrial Fibrillation
- Heart Failure: Beta-blocker Therapy
- CAD: Beta-blocker Therapy for CAD Patients with prior MI
- CAD: Drug Therapy for Lowering LDL
- CAD: Oral Antiplatelet Therapy for CAD Patients
- Ischemic Vascular Disease: Blood Pressure Management
- Ischemic Vascular Disease: Use of Aspirin or other Antithrombotics
- Ischemic Vascular Disease: Complete Lipid Panel and LDL Control
- Controlling High Blood Pressure

CQM MENU SET (9 OF 38) DIABETES

- Diabetes: Hemoglobin A1c
- Diabetes: LDL Management
- Diabetes: Blood Pressure Management
- Diabetes: Hemoglobin A1c Control (less than 8.0%)
- Diabetes: Eye Exam
- Diabetes: Urine Screening
- Diabetes: Foot Exam
- Diabetic Retinopathy: Presence of Macular Edema and Retinopathy Severity
- Diabetic Retinopathy: Communication with Physician Managing Ongoing Care

CQM MENU SET (6 OF 38) ONCOLOGY

- Breast Cancer: Screening
- Breast Cancer: Hormonal Therapy for Stage IC-IIIC Estrogen Receptor Positive
- Colorectal Cancer: Screening
- Colon Cancer: Chemotherapy for Stage III Patients
- Cervical Cancer: Screening
- Prostate Cancer: Avoidance of Bone Scan Overuse for Staging Low-risk Prostate Cancer

CQM MENU SET (3 OF 38) ASTHMA

- Asthma Pharmacologic Therapy
- Asthma Assessment
- Use of Appropriate Medications for Asthma

CQM MENU SET (3 OF 38) INFECTIOUS

- Chlamydia Screening for Women
- Pneumonia Vaccine Status of their Patients
- Testing for Children with Pharyngitis

CQM MENU SET (3 OF 38) DEPENDENCIES

- Smoking and Tobacco use Cessation: Counseling for Cessation Strategies
- Initiation and Engagement of Alcohol and other Drug Dependence Treatments
- Antidepressant Medication Management

CQM MENU SET (2 OF 38) PRENATAL CARE

- Prenatal Care: Screening for HIV
- Prenatal Care: Anti-D Immune Globulin

CQM MENU SET (1 OF 38) GLAUCOMA

- Primary Open Angle Glaucoma: Optic Nerve Evaluation

CQM MENU SET (1 OF 38) LOW BACK PAIN

- Appropriate use of Imaging Studies

As with the core set and menu set measures, there are certain CQMs that are more likely to be relevant to certain medical professionals than others. EPs are required to select three core/alternate core CQMs in addition to three selections from the discretionary set. If an EP reports zeros for one or more of the required core CQMs, they must then report on up to three alternate core CQMs.

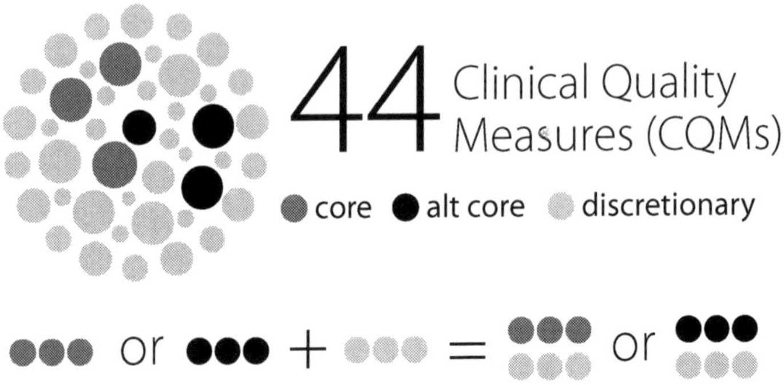

Note: In 2012 and 2013, Stage 1 CQM reporting may be conducted via Attestation (**attestation.theMUguide.com**) or eReporting Pilot (**ereporting.theMUguide.com**). Starting in 2014, all Medicare EPs must submit CQM data via Attestation in their first year and, in subsequent years, must electronically submit CQM data to CMS.

2014+: Clinical Quality Measures (CQMs)

Beginning in 2014, new CQMs, which apply to all providers regardless of program stage, go into effect in order to better align with Health and Human Services (HHS) priorities. EPs in their first year of the program must report CQMs by attestation because it is the only reporting method that would allow them to meet submission deadlines to avoid payment adjustments. Beyond their first year, Medicare EPs have several individual and group CQM reporting options to choose from.

CQM Reporting Option (Individual): Aggregate Reporting through CMS-designated Electronic Transmission using CEHRT

For Medicare EPs, each individual provider will be required to report on 9 out of 64 CQMs. Providers are free to choose those CQMs that provide most value to their practice and patient care, but all EPs are required to select at least three (3) CQMs from the following six (6) National Quality Strategy domains:

- Patient/Family Engagement (4 of 64 CQMs)
- Patient Safety (6 of 64 CQMs)
- Care Coordination (1 of 64 CQMs)
- Population/Public Health (9 of 64 CQMs)
- Efficient Use of Healthcare Resources (4 of 64 CQMs)
- Clinical Processes/Effectiveness (40 of 64 CQMs)

Note: If no CQMs are applicable to the EP's scope of practice and patient population, the EP must report "zeros" for 9 CQMs.

CQM Reporting Option (Individual): Physician Quality Reporting System (PQRS) EHR Reporting Option

Individual EPs have the option to report CQMs under the PQRS EHR Reporting Option using CEHRT. Please refer to 42 CFR §414.90 and the CY2013 Medicare PFS proposed rule (77 FR 44988) for more information.

CQM Reporting Option (Group): Medicare Shared Savings Program (SSP)

Medicare EPs participating in the Medicare SSP and the testing of the Pioneer Accountable Care Organization (ACO) model who use CEHRT to submit ACO measures in accordance with the requirements of the Medicare SSP would be considered to have satisfied their CQM reporting requirement as a group for the Medicare EHR Incentive Program.

Note: EPs who use this group option would be required to comply with any changes to the Medicare SSP that may apply in the future.

CQM Reporting Option (Group): Physician Quality Reporting System (PQRS) Group Practice Reporting Option

Medicare EPs who satisfactorily report PQRS CQMs using CEHRT under the PQRS Group Practice Reporting Option (GPRO), would be considered to have satisfied their CQM reporting requirement as a group for the Medicare EHR Incentive Program.

Note: EPs who use this group option would be required to comply with any changes to the PQRS GPRO that may apply in the future.

The following is a list of the 64 CQMs available for reporting beginning in 2014.

Note: An asterisk (*) indicates new CY2014 CQMs.

Stay Up-to-Date: A designation of "TBD" below means that a measure has not yet been endorsed as of the time of writing. For updates related to CQM endorsements, go to **cqms.theMUguide.com**.

CQM CY2014 (4 OF 64) PATIENT/FAMILY ENGAGEMENT

- Functional Status Assessment for Complex Chronic Conditions (TBD)*
- Functional Status Assessment for Knee Replacement (TBD)*
- Functional Status Assessment for Hip Replacement (TBD)*
- Oncology: Medical and Radiation—Pain Intensity Quantified (NQF 0384)*

CQM CY2014 (6 OF 64) PATIENT SAFETY

- ADE Prevention and Monitoring: Warfarin Time in Therapeutic Range (TBD)*
- Child and Adolescent Major Depressive Disorder: Suicide Risk Assessment (NQF 1365)*
- Use of High-Risk Medications in the Elderly (NQF 0022)*
- Documentation of Current Medications in the Medical Record (NQF 0419)*
- Cataracts: Complications within 30 days Following Cataract Surgery Requiring Additional Surgical Procedures (NQF 0564)*
- Falls: Screening for Future Fall Risk (NQF 0101)*

CQM CY2014 (1 OF 64) CARE COORDINATION

- Closing the Referral Loop: Receipt of Specialist Report (TBD)*

CQM CY2014 (9 OF 64) POPULATION/ PUBLIC HEALTH

- Preventive Care and Screening: Screening for High Blood Pressure and Follow-Up Documented (TBD)*
- Preventive Care and Screening: Screening for Clinical Depression and Follow-Up Plan (NQF 0418)*
- Maternal Depression Screening (NQF 1401)*
- Chlamydia Screening for Women (NQF 0033)
- Preventive Care and Screening: Tobacco Use: Screening and Cessation Intervention (NQF 0028)
- Childhood Immunization Status (NQF 0038)
- Preventive Care and Screening: Influenza Immunization (NQF 0041)
- Preventive Care and Screening: Body Mass Index (BMI) Screening and Follow-Up (NQF 0421)
- Weight Assessment and Counseling for Nutrition and Physical Activity for Children and Adolescents (NQF 0024)

CQM CY2014 (4 OF 64) EFFICIENT USE OF HEALTHCARE RESOURCES

- Appropriate Treatment for Children with Upper Respiratory Infection (URI) (NQF 0069)*
- Use of Imaging Studies for Low Back Pain (NQF 0052)
- Appropriate Testing for Children with Pharyngitis (NQF 0002)
- Prostate Cancer: Avoidance of Overuse of Bone Scan for Staging Low Risk Prostate Cancer Patients (NQF 0389)

CQM CY2014 (40 OF 64) CLINICAL PROCESSES/EFFECTIVENESS

- Preventive Care and Screening: Cholesterol—Fasting Low Density Lipoprotein (LDL-C) Test Performed (TBD)*
- Preventive Care and Screening: Risk-stratified Cholesterol—Fasting Low Density Lipoprotein (LDL-C) (TBD)*
- Hypertension: Improvement in Blood Pressure (TBD)*
- HIV/AIDS: Medical Visit (NQF 0403)*
- HIV/AIDS: Pneumocystis Jiroveci Pneumonia (PCP) Prophylaxis (NQF 0405)*
- HIV/AIDS: RNA Control for Patients with HIV (TBD)*
- Children who have Dental Decay or Cavities (TBD)*
- Primary Caries Prevention Intervention as Offered by Primary Care Providers, including Dentists (TBD)*
- Major Depressive Disorder (MDD): Suicide Risk Assessment (NQF 0104)*
- ADHD: Follow-Up Care for Children Prescribed Attention-Deficit/Hyperactivity Disorder (ADHD) Medication (NQF 0108)*
- Bipolar Disorder and Major Depression: Appraisal for Alcohol or Chemical Substance Use (NQF 0110)*
- Depression Remission at Twelve Months (NQF 0710)*
- Depression Utilization of the PHQ-9 Tool (NQF 0712)*
- Dementia: Cognitive Assessment (TBD)*
- Pregnant Women that had HBsAg Testing (NQF 0608)*
- Cataracts: 20/40 or Better Visual Acuity within 90 Days Following Cataract Surgery (NQF 0565)*
- Heart Failure (HF): Angiotensin-Converting Enzyme (ACE) Inhibitor or Angiotensin Receptor Blocker (ARB) Therapy for Left Ventricular Systolic Dysfunction (LVSD) (NQF 0081)
- Heart Failure (HF): Beta-Blocker Therapy for Left Ventricular Systolic Dysfunction (LVSD) (NQF 0083)
- Coronary Artery Disease (CAD): Beta-Blocker Therapy - Prior Myocardial Infarction (MI) or Left Ventricular Systolic Dysfunction (LVEF <40%) (NQF 0070)
- Ischemic Vascular Disease (IVD): Use of Aspirin or another Antithrombotic (NQF 0068)
- Ischemic Vascular Disease (IVD): Complete Lipid Panel and LDL Control (NQF 0075)
- Controlling High Blood Pressure (NQF 0018)
- Diabetes: Hemoglobin A1c Poor Control (NQF 0059)
- Diabetes: Hemoglobin A1c Test for Pediatric Patients (NQF 0060)
- Diabetes: Low Density Lipoprotein (LDL) Management (NQF 0064)
- Diabetes: Eye Exam (NQF 0055)

- Diabetes: Urine Protein Screening (NQF 0062)
- Diabetes: Foot Exam (NQF 0056)
- Diabetic Retinopathy: Documentation of Presence or Absence of Macular Edema and Level of Severity of Retinopathy (NQF 0088)
- Diabetic Retinopathy: Communication with the Physician Managing Ongoing Diabetes Care (NQF 0089)
- Pneumonia Vaccination Status for Older Adults (NQF 0043)
- Breast Cancer Screening (NQF 0031)
- Breast Cancer: Hormonal Therapy for Stage IC-IIIC Estrogen Receptor/Progesterone Receptor (ER/PR) Positive Breast Cancer (NQF 0387)
- Colorectal Cancer Screening (NQF 0034)
- Colon Cancer: Chemotherapy for AJCC Stage III Colon Cancer Patients (NQF 0385)
- Cervical Cancer Screening (NQF 0032)
- Initiation and Engagement of Alcohol and Other Drug Dependence Treatment (NQF 0004)
- Anti-depressant Medication Management (NQF 0105)
- Use of Appropriate Medications for Asthma (NQF 0036)
- Primary Open Angle Glaucoma (POAG): Optic Nerve Evaluation (NQF 0086)

Stay Up-to-Date: Under certain circumstances, CMS may potentially remove specific CQMs. Also, CMS has published a set of nine (9) recommended CQMs for both adult and pediatric populations. For the latest information about CQM changes as well as recommended CQMs, go to **cqms.theMUguide.com**.

You will need to assess each individual EP in your group and select the CQMs that are most relevant and applicable to your provider and patient population.

Part I:

STAGE 1 OBJECTIVES AND MEASURES

CHAPTER 4

Policies, Guidelines, and Audits

Learn more about policies, guidelines, and audits.

To access more information about group policies and audits, scan the QR code above or go to **policies.theMUguide.com**.

In this chapter, we help identify and define policies that will assist you with documenting your action plans and MU strategy as they relate to workload reductions. We also briefly touch upon considerations related to risks, audits, and record keeping.

Developing and implementing a set of well-defined group policies provides a solid foundation when it comes to addressing workload reduction opportunities as part of your MU strategy. Moreover, creating standard policies for various activities yields a set of documented interpretations of the regulations as you see fit for your individual practice. This activity also brings consistency across practices and provides a safe harbor.

Now, let's examine the set of policies that your practice may choose to adopt.

Stage 2 Final Rule Impact: Stage 2 Final Rules introduced a number changes or updates to some of the Stage 1 criteria. An asterisk (*) on the following pages indicates a change notice for those specific Stage 1 criteria. Please refer to the core, menu, and CQM criteria in Chapters 1, 2 and 3 for specific details.

"Seen by the EP" Policy

The purpose of this policy is to create documentation that might allow for a potential reduction of the patient population used for the denominator of all related objectives and measures. In order to realize this opportunity, the CEHRT used by the EP must be able to accommodate a separate denominator for the associated measures (consult with your CEHRT provider regarding this capability).

In the first year of the program, CMS published guidance (refer to CMS FAQ#3307/FAQ#3309) that might enhance the ability for certain physicians to comply with meaningful use program requirements. The verbiage "seen by the EP" originally implied that any service rendered by the EP, should be included in final meaningful use measure calculations. The implication of this guidance released by

CMS indicates that an EP who performs diagnostic activities only, could conceivably choose to limit their "seen" patients to physical visits, omitting telemedicine and similar services with minimal consultative service for the patient, for meaningful use measures that include "seen by the EP" verbiage (patient populations must be ≥1).

While there is flexibility in this language, CMS does require that the EP have a consistent policy on when to include or omit these patients from their calculations. In addition, a secondary FAQ was published indicating that when a patient is seen by the EP's clinical staff and not the EP themselves, the EP can elect to include or not include those patients in their meaningful use calculations as long as the decision applies universally to all patients across the required measures. The following Stage 1 criteria are associated with this policy:

CORE SET

- **42 CFR §495.6(d)(1):** Use computerized provider order entry (CPOE) for medication orders directly entered by any licensed health care professional who can enter orders into the medical record per state, local, and professional guidelines*
- **42 CFR §495.6(d)(3):** Maintain an up-to-date problem list of current and active diagnoses
- **42 CFR §495.6(d)(5):** Maintain active medication list
- **42 CFR §495.6(d)(6):** Maintain active medication allergy list
- **42 CFR §495.6(d)(7):** Record demographics: preferred language, gender, race, ethnicity, date of birth
- **42 CFR §495.6(d)(8):** Record and chart changes in vital signs: height, weight, blood pressure. Calculate and display BMI, plot and display growth charts for children 2–20 years (including BMI)*
- **42 CFR §495.6(d)(9):** Record smoking status for patients 13 years old or older
- **42 CFR §495.6(d)(12):** Provide patients with an electronic copy of their health information (including diagnostic test results, problem list, medication lists, medication allergies) upon request* (effective 2014, a new measure introduces "Seen by the EP" verbiage for this objective)

MENU SET

- **42 CFR §495.6(e)(5):** Provide patients with timely electronic access to their health information (including lab results, problem list, medication lists, medication allergies) within four business days of the information being available to the EP*
- **42 CFR §495.6(e)(6):** Use certified EHR technology to identify patient-specific education resources and provide those resources to the patient if appropriate

Note: Many providers have found it helpful to add a "Seen by the EP" and "Office Visit" designation to their Charge Master to identify procedures that encompass face-to-face encounters. By making these designations, it becomes an easier, and well documented, method for determining which EPs in your practice qualify for the "Seen by the EP" policy, should you choose to adopt it.

"Office Visit" Policy

The purpose of this policy is to create documentation that might allow for a potential reduction of the patient population used for the denominator of all related objectives and measures. In order to realize this opportunity, the CEHRT used by the EP must be able to accommodate a separate denominator for the associated measures (consult with your CEHRT provider regarding this capability).

According to the regulatory definition, office visits include separate, billable encounters that result from evaluation and management services provided to the patient and include: (1) concurrent care or transfer of care visits, (2) consultant visits, or (3) prolonged physician service without direct (face-to-face) patient contact (tele-health). A consultant visit occurs when a provider is asked to render an expert opinion/service for a specific condition or problem by a referring provider. CMS asserts that there is room for discretion in the definition (e.g. 'office visit' is not limited to E&M services) and the most important consideration in utilizing this discretion is that the policy applies for the entire reporting period and across all patients. The following Stage 1 criteria are associated with this policy:

CORE SET

- **42 CFR §495.6(d)(13):** Provide clinical summaries for patients for each office visit

Note: Related objectives and measures for this policy will change in Stage 2 as many more objective level measures and exclusions incorporate the concept of 'office visits.'

"Vital Sign" Policy

The purpose of this policy is to create documentation that might allow for a potential exclusion based on what vital signs the EP considers relevant to scope of practice. According to the regulatory definition, the vital sign exclusion may apply to any EP who either sees no patients 2 years or older, or who believes that all three vital signs of height, weight, and blood pressure have no relevance to their scope of practice. Effective in 2013, any EP who believes that height and weight are relevant to their scope of practice, but not blood pressure, may be excluded from recording blood pressure. The following Stage 1 criteria are associated with this policy:

CORE SET

- **42 CFR §495.6(d)(8):** Record and chart changes in vital signs: height, weight, blood pressure. Calculate and display BMI, plot and display growth charts for children 2–20 years (including BMI)*

"Medication Order" Policy

The purpose of this policy is to create documentation that might allow for a potential exclusion based on how you define supplies (e.g. authorizations for items/supplies such as durable medical equipment and contrast agents) from other pharmaceuticals that are considered medications. In order to claim an exclusion, EPs need to demonstrate the ability to order less than 100 medications during the EHR reporting period. The following Stage 1 criteria are associated with this policy:

CORE SET

- **42 CFR §495.6(d)(1):** Use computerized provider order entry (CPOE) for medication orders directly entered by any licensed health care professional who can enter orders into the medical record per state, local, and professional guidelines*
- **42 CFR §495.6(d)(4):** Generate and transmit permissible prescriptions electronically (eRx)*

MENU SET

- **42 CFR §495.6(e)(1):** Implement drug-formulary checks

"Lab Order" Policy

The purpose of this policy is to create documentation that might allow for a potential exclusion based on laboratory exams ordered by the EP, namely, less than 100 exams that result in numeric and/or positive/negative results. The following Stage 1 criteria are associated with this policy:

MENU SET

- **42 CFR §495.6(e)(2):** Incorporate clinical lab test results into certified EHR technology as structured data

"CQM Selection" Policy

The purpose for this policy is to describe which CQMs were chosen for reporting by the EP and why they were selected. Prior to 2014, this includes demonstrating a total of 6 out of 44 CQMs (three core/alternate core measures and three discretionary measures). Beginning in 2014, this includes reporting 9 out of 64 CQMs (selected from at least 3 out of 6 National Quality Strategy domains). If no CQMs are applicable to the EP's scope of practice and patient population, the EP must report "zeros" and should include record of this decision in their policy documentation. The following Stage 1 criteria are associated with this policy:

CORE SET

- **42 CFR §495.6(d)(10):** Report ambulatory clinical quality measures to CMS or the States*

"Clinical Decision Support" Policy

The purpose of this policy is to record justification as to why the EP has selected their chosen CDS rules. Federal regulation states that EPs need to implement CDS that is relevant to specialty or high clinical priority, but if an EP's CEHRT only offers limited alternatives, the EP should state why the chosen CDS was used to meet the associated objectives. CMS will not issue additional guidance on the selection of appropriate clinical decision support rules for Stage 1 Meaningful Use. This determination is best left to the EP taking into account their workflow, patient population, and quality improvement efforts. Also, drug-drug and drug-allergy interaction alerts cannot be used to meet the meaningful use objective for implementing one clinical decision support rule. EPs must implement one clinical decision support rule in addition to drug-drug and drug-allergy interaction checks. The following Stage 1 criteria are associated with this policy:

CORE SET

- **42 CFR §495.6(d)(11):** Implement one clinical decision support rule relevant to specialty or high clinical priority along with the ability to track compliance with that rule

"Patient Request" Policy

The purpose of this policy is to define how EPs monitor the request from patients for their health information. An EP may withhold information from the electronic copy of a patient's health information in accordance with the HIPAA Privacy Rule (specified at 45 CFR §164.524). If an EP works in an environment where there are no patient requests (e.g. telemedicine settings), the EP should state that reasoning in preparation for exclusion from this measure. Lastly, this policy can be used to determine the denominator for measure related thresholds. The following Stage 1 criteria are associated with this policy:

CORE SET

- **42 CFR §495.6(d)(12):** Provide patients with an electronic copy of their health information (including diagnostic test results, problem list, medication lists, medication allergies) upon request*

"Information Exchange Methodology" Policy

For EPs reporting in 2012, this policy should reflect the exact method used to demonstrate compliance. EPs can use their clinical judgment to identify what clinical information is considered key clinical information for purposes of exchanging clinical information about a patient at a particular time with other providers of care. Simulated transfers of information are not acceptable, but an unsuccessful test of electronic exchange of key clinical information will be considered valid for meeting the measure of the objective related to this policy. Effective 2013, the Stage 1 criteria related to this policy has been removed in favor of the more robust, actual use case of electronic exchange through a summary of care record following each transition of care or referral. The following Stage 1 criteria are associated with this policy:

CORE SET

- **42 CFR §495.6(d)(14):** Capability to exchange key clinical information (for example: problem list, medication list, medication allergies, diagnostic test results) among providers of care and patient authorized entities electronically*

"Security Risk Analysis Methodology" Policy

This policy should describe the exact security risk analysis method used to demonstrate compliance, including the date of conduct or review, and all parties involved in performing the analysis. EPs must conduct or review a security risk analysis of CEHRT and implement updates as necessary at least once prior to the end of each EHR reporting period and attest to that conduct or review. If the method changes for different reporting periods, these changes should be recorded in the policy. The following Stage 1 criteria are associated with this policy:

CORE SET

- **42 CFR §495.6(d)(15):** Protect electronic health information created or maintained by the certified EHR technology through the implementation of appropriate technical capabilities

"Patient List" Policy

The EP is best positioned to determine which reports are most useful to their care efforts (quality improvement, reduction of disparities, research, or outreach), and therefore, this policy should describe the exact purpose of the list(s) created. EPs must generate these lists for each EHR reporting period. If the reports change for different reporting periods, these changes should be recorded in the policy. The policy should also include the date performed as well as who generated the list. The following Stage 1 criteria are associated with this policy:

MENU SET

- **42 CFR §495.6(e)(3):** Generate lists of patients by specific conditions to use for quality improvement, reduction of disparities, research, or outreach

"Patient Age" Policy

The purpose of this policy is to create documentation that might allow for a potential exclusion based on the age of all patients. If an EP can demonstrate through CEHRT records that they have no patients 65 years or older, or 5 years or younger, than they can be excluded from the criteria related to this policy. The following Stage 1 criteria are associated with this policy:

MENU SET

- **42 CFR §495.6(e)(4):** Send reminders to patients per patient preference for preventive/follow-up care

"Physician Discretion" Policy

The purpose of this policy is to formulate and record a strategic methodology for patient access to their health information, which may be subject to the discretion of the EP to withhold certain information. The justification of such withholdings may be formulated on a case-by-case or exam level basis, but should be documented and retained. The following Stage 1 criteria are associated with this policy:

CORE SET

- **42 CFR §495.6(d)(12):** Provide patients with an electronic copy of their health information (including diagnostic test results, problem list, medication lists, medication allergies) upon request*

MENU SET

- **42 CFR §495.6(e)(5):** Provide patients with timely electronic access to their health information (including lab results, problem list, medication lists, medication allergies) within four business days of the information being available to the EP*

"Transitions of Care" Policy

The purpose of this policy is to create documentation that might allow for a potential exclusion based on the definition and use of transition of care into, and referrals or transfers out of, an EP's practice. The following Stage 1 criteria are associated with this policy:

MENU SET

- **42 CFR §495.6(e)(7):** The EP who receives a patient from another setting of care or provider of care or believes an encounter is relevant should perform medication reconciliation
- **42 CFR §495.6(e)(8):** The EP who transitions their patient to another setting of care or refers their patient to another provider of care should provide summary of care record for each transition of care or referral

"Immunization Administration" Policy

The purpose of this policy is to create documentation that might allow for a potential exclusion based on the absence of administration of immunizations in an EP's practice. If multiple EPs use the same CEHRT in a shared physical setting, testing would only have to occur once for a given certified technology. The transmission of actual patient information is not required for the purposes of a test and an unsuccessful test is considered valid and would satisfy the criteria related to this policy. Lastly, the transmission of immunization information must use the standards at 45 CFR §170.302(k). The following Stage 1 criteria are associated with this policy:

MENU SET

- **42 CFR §495.6(e)(9):** Capability to submit electronic data to immunization registries or Immunization Information Systems and actual submission in accordance with applicable law and practice*

"Syndromic Surveillance" Policy

The purpose of this policy is to create documentation that might allow for a potential exclusion based on the absence of the collection of syndromic information in an EP's practice. If multiple EPs use the same CEHRT in a shared physical setting, testing would only have to occur once for a given certified technology. The transmission of electronic syndromic surveillance data is not required for the purposes of a test and an unsuccessful test is considered valid and would satisfy the criteria related to this policy. Lastly, the transmission of syndromic surveillance information must use the standards at 45 CFR §170.302(l). The following Stage 1 criteria are associated with this policy:

MENU SET

- **42 CFR §495.6(e)(10):** Capability to submit electronic syndromic surveillance data to public health agencies and actual submission in accordance with applicable law and practice*

Risks, audits, and record keeping

According to documentation in the CMS Stage 1 Final Rule, one commenter expressed a concern that "attestation is an insufficient means to hold providers accountable for the expenditure of public funds and to protect against fraud and abuse." CMS shares the concern for potential fraud and abuse and has developed an audit strategy to address these types of risks. With that said, any EP attesting to receive an incentive payment under the program may be subject to an audit by the government.

While there are some requirements, like the fact that providers participating in the incentive programs must retain all documentation that supports their demonstration of meaningful use for six years after attestation, EPs can do more to prepare by managing the additional risks associated with attestation. Aside from retaining paper and electronic versions of core and menu set records, cost reports, payment calculations, and CQM documentation, your organization can implement a formal risk analysis process, follow existing security and privacy standards, as well as demonstrate due diligence in risk identification and implementation.

The government has already started conducting audits on health care providers that have received payments under the CMS EHR Incentive Programs. If your organization is the subject of an audit, you will be required to provide, but not limited to, (1) proof that you are using CEHRT, (2) documentation supporting your core set objectives and measures attestation, and (3) documentation supporting your menu set objectives and measures attestation.

Stay Up-to-Date: For the latest information about CMS EHR Incentive Program audits, go to **audits.theMUguide.com**.

Part I:

STAGE 1 OBJECTIVES AND MEASURES

CHAPTER 5

Criteria Level Exclusions

Find out more about criteria level exclusions.

To review criteria level exclusions online, obtain access to program updates, and review specifications related to EPs, scan the QR code above or go to **stage1exclusions.theMUguide.com**.

In this chapter, we examine a variety of exclusionary considerations by taking a look at specific Stage 1 criteria grouped by exclusion availability, provider activities, and attestation requirements.

In addition to establishing group policies, it is important to analyze individual criteria and assess exclusion opportunities for those criteria not covered by group policies. The following lists represent those criteria with no exclusions, those with exclusion opportunities available, exclusion opportunities based on diagnostic activities, and methods for calculating measures.

Stage 2 Final Rule Impact: Stage 2 Final Rules introduced a number changes or updates to some of the Stage 1 criteria. An asterisk (*) indicates a change notice for those specific Stage 1 criteria. Please refer to the core, menu, and CQM criteria in Chapters 1, 2 and 3 for specific details.

No Criteria-level Exclusion

The following is a list of all Stage 1 criteria that lack exclusion opportunities. In other words, all EPs are required to report on these criteria.

CORE SET

- **42 CFR §495.6(d)(2):** Implement drug-drug and drug-allergy interaction checks
- **42 CFR §495.6(d)(3):** Maintain an up-to-date problem list of current and active diagnoses
- **42 CFR §495.6(d)(5):** Maintain active medication list
- **42 CFR §495.6(d)(6):** Maintain active medication allergy list
- **42 CFR §495.6(d)(7):** Record demographics: preferred language, gender, race, ethnicity, date of birth
- **42 CFR §495.6(d)(10):** Report ambulatory clinical quality measures to CMS or the States*
- **42 CFR §495.6(d)(11):** Implement one clinical decision support rule relevant to specialty or high clinical priority along with the ability to track compliance with that rule
- **42 CFR §495.6(d)(14):** Capability to exchange key clinical information (for example: problem list, medication list, medication allergies, diagnostic test results) among providers of care and patient authorized entities electronically*
- **42 CFR §495.6(d)(15):** Protect electronic health information created or maintained by the certified EHR technology through the implementation of appropriate technical capabilities

MENU SET

- **42 CFR §495.6(e)(3):** Generate lists of patients by specific conditions to use for quality improvement, reduction of disparities, research, or outreach
- **42 CFR §495.6(e)(6):** Use certified EHR technology to identify patient-specific education resources and provide those resources to the patient if appropriate

Criteria-level Exclusion Available

The following is a list of all Stage 1 criteria that have exclusion opportunities available.

CORE SET

- **42 CFR §495.6(d)(1):** Use computerized provider order entry (CPOE) for medication orders directly entered by any licensed health care professional who can enter orders into the medical record per state, local, and professional guidelines*
- **42 CFR §495.6(d)(4):** Generate and transmit permissible prescriptions electronically (eRx)*
- **42 CFR §495.6(d)(8):** Record and chart changes in vital signs: height, weight, blood pressure. Calculate and display BMI, plot and display growth charts for children 2–20 years (including BMI)*
- **42 CFR §495.6(d)(9):** Record smoking status for patients 13 years old or older
- **42 CFR §495.6(d)(12):** Provide patients with an electronic copy of their health information (including diagnostic test results, problem list, medication lists, medication allergies) upon request*
- **42 CFR §495.6(d)(13):** Provide clinical summaries for patients for each office visit

MENU SET

- **42 CFR §495.6(e)(1):** Implement drug-formulary checks
- **42 CFR §495.6(e)(2):** Incorporate clinical lab test results into certified EHR technology as structured data
- **42 CFR §495.6(e)(4):** Send reminders to patients per patient preference for preventive/follow-up care
- **42 CFR §495.6(e)(5):** Provide patients with timely electronic access to their health information (including lab results, problem list, medication lists, medication allergies) within four business days of the information being available to the EP*
- **42 CFR §495.6(e)(7):** The EP who receives a patient from another setting of care or provider of care or believes an encounter is relevant should perform medication reconciliation
- **42 CFR §495.6(e)(8):** The EP who transitions their patient to another setting of care or refers their patient to another provider of care should provide summary of care record for each transition of care or referral

- **42 CFR §495.6(e)(9):** Capability to submit electronic data to immunization registries or Immunization Information Systems and actual submission in accordance with applicable law and practice*
- **42 CFR §495.6(e)(10):** Capability to submit electronic syndromic surveillance data to public health agencies and actual submission in accordance with applicable law and practice*

Note: The following exclusion opportunities are only samples for providers based on activities performed. You will need to analyze each EP in your practice in order to fully determine the final set of core and menu set criteria required to achieve meaningful use.

Potential exclusion opportunities based on diagnostic activities

Now, let's examine the potential set of criteria required for EPs who perform diagnostic activities with no procedural activities. The list below outlines potential core and menu set objectives up for consideration based on individual activities performed, after exemptions are taken. Keep in mind that workload may further be reduced with group policies (refer to Chapter 4 for more information about group policies).

CORE SET

- **42 CFR §495.6(d)(2):** Implement drug-drug and drug-allergy interaction checks
- **42 CFR §495.6(d)(3):** Maintain an up-to-date problem list of current and active diagnoses ("Seen by the EP" measure; see Chapter 4 for policy guidance)
- **42 CFR §495.6(d)(5):** Maintain active medication list ("Seen by the EP" measure; see Chapter 4 for policy guidance)
- **42 CFR §495.6(d)(6):** Maintain active medication allergy list ("Seen by the EP" measure; see Chapter 4 for policy guidance)
- **42 CFR §495.6(d)(7):** Record demographics (preferred language, gender, race, ethnicity, date of birth) ("Seen by the EP" measure; see Chapter 4 for policy guidance)
- **42 CFR §495.6(d)(9):** Record smoking status for patients 13 years old or older ("Seen by the EP" measure; see Chapter 4 for policy guidance)
- **42 CFR §495.6(d)(10):** Report ambulatory clinical quality measures to CMS or the States*
- **42 CFR §495.6(d)(11):** Implement one clinical decision support rule relevant to specialty or high clinical priority along with the ability to track compliance with that rule

- **42 CFR §495.6(d)(12):** Provide patients with an electronic copy of their health information (including diagnostic test results, problem list, medication list, medication allergies) upon request* (effective 2014, a new measure introduces "Seen by the EP" verbiage for this objective; see Chapter 4 for policy guidance)
- **42 CFR §495.6(d)(14):** Capability to exchange key clinical information (for example: problem list, medication list, medication allergies, diagnostic test results) among providers of care and patient-authorized entities electronically*
- **42 CFR §495.6(d)(15):** Protect electronic health information created or maintained by the certified EHR technology through the implementation of appropriate technical capabilities

MENU SET

- **42 CFR §495.6(e)(3):** Generate lists of patients by specific conditions to use for quality improvement, reduction of disparities, research or outreach
- **42 CFR §495.6(e)(4):** Send reminders to patients per patient preference for preventive/follow-up care
- **42 CFR §495.6(e)(5):** Provide patients with timely electronic access to their health information (including lab results, problem list, medication list, medication allergies) within four business days of the information being available to the EP* ("Seen by the EP" measure; see Chapter 4 for policy guidance)
- **42 CFR §495.6(e)(6):** Use certified EHR technology to identify patient-specific education resources and provide those resources to the patient if appropriate ("Seen by the EP" measure; see Chapter 4 for policy guidance)

CLINICAL QUALITY MEASURES: Medicare EPs are also required to report clinical quality measures (CQMs). Prior to 2014, EPs are required to demonstrate and report a total of 6 out of 44 clinical quality measures: 3 core/alternate core measures and 3 discretionary measures from the remaining 38 measures. Beginning in 2014, providers will be required to report on 9 out of 64 CQMs (refer to Chapter 3 for more information about CQMs).

Methods for Calculating Measures

For EPs, there are a few ways of measuring compliance based on calculation requirements for each specific core and menu set objective. The three types of reporting requirements include measures with a denominator of unique patients regardless of whether the patient's records are maintained using certified EHR technology, measures with a denominator based on counting actions for patients whose records are maintained using certified EHR technology, and measures requiring only a yes/no attestation.

The following objectives have associated measures with a denominator of unique patients regardless of whether the patient's records are maintained using CEHRT:

- **42 CFR §495.6(d)(3):** Maintain an up-to-date problem list of current and active diagnoses
- **42 CFR §495.6(d)(5):** Maintain active medication list
- **42 CFR §495.6(d)(6):** Maintain active medication allergy list
- **42 CFR §495.6(d)(7):** Record demographics: preferred language, gender, race, ethnicity, date of birth
- **42 CFR §495.6(e)(5):** Provide patients with timely electronic access to their health information (including lab results, problem list, medication list, medication allergies) within four business days of the information being available to the EP*
- **42 CFR §495.6(e)(6):** Use certified EHR technology to identify patient-specific education resources and provide those resources to the patient if appropriate

The following objectives have associated measures with a denominator based on counting actions for patients whose records are maintained using CEHRT:

- **42 CFR §495.6(d)(1):** Use computerized provider order entry (CPOE) for medication orders directly entered by any licensed health care professional who can enter orders into the medical record per state, local, and professional guidelines*
- **42 CFR §495.6(d)(4):** Generate and transmit permissible prescriptions electronically (eRx)*
- **42 CFR §495.6(d)(8):** Record and chart changes in vital signs: height, weight, blood pressure. Calculate and display BMI, plot and display growth charts for children 2–20 years (including BMI)*
- **42 CFR §495.6(d)(9):** Record smoking status for patients 13 years old or older
- **42 CFR §495.6(d)(12):** Provide patients with an electronic copy of their health information (including diagnostic test results, problem list, medication list, medication allergies) upon request*
- **42 CFR §495.6(d)(13):** Provide clinical summaries for patients for each office visit
- **42 CFR §495.6(e)(2):** Incorporate clinical lab test results into certified EHR technology as structured data
- **42 CFR §495.6(e)(4):** Send reminders to patients per patient preference for preventive/follow-up care
- **42 CFR §495.6(e)(7):** The EP who receives a patient from another setting of care or provider of care or believes an encounter is relevant should perform medication reconciliation

- **42 CFR §495.6(e)(8):** The EP who transitions their patient to another setting of care or provider of care or refers their patient to another provider of care should provide summary of care record for each transition of care or referral

The following objectives have associated measures requiring only a yes/no attestation:

- **42 CFR §495.6(d)(2):** Implement drug-drug and drug-allergy interaction checks
- **42 CFR §495.6(d)(11):** Implement one clinical decision support rule relevant to specialty or high clinical priority along with the ability to track compliance with that rule
- **42 CFR §495.6(d)(14):** Capability to exchange key clinical information (for example: problem list, medication list, medication allergies, diagnostic test results) among providers of care and patient-authorized entities electronically*
- **42 CFR §495.6(d)(15):** Protect electronic health information created or maintained by the certified EHR technology through the implementation of appropriate technical capabilities
- **42 CFR §495.6(e)(1):** Implement drug-formulary checks
- **42 CFR §495.6(e)(3):** Generate lists of patients by specific conditions to use for quality improvement, reduction of disparities, research or outreach
- **42 CFR §495.6(e)(9):** Capability to submit electronic data to immunization registries or Immunization Information Systems and actual submission in accordance with applicable law and practice*
- **42 CFR §495.6(e)(10):** Capability to submit electronic syndromic surveillance data to public health agencies and actual submission in accordance with applicable law and practice*

These measure-type groups were designed to reduce the burden on providers. For more information about the various types of measure groupings, refer to the incentive programs Final Rule (FR 75 44376 – 44380).

Consistency is key here. Once you've defined your exclusion activities and group policies, you should create a comprehensive set of compliance records that explicitly document your organization's specific MU policies, measures and exclusions, participants, and workflow strategy. Upon completion, you should review these final MU compliance documents with your institutional stakeholders, including, but not limited to, your CMO, CIO, MU implementation teams, and general counsel. Lastly, it's suggested that you review these documents with departmental stakeholders before implementing your strategy.

Part II:

BEYOND STAGE 1 MU

In Part II, we take a look at Stage 2 Meaningful Use and the impact that the Stage 2 Final Rules have on Stage 1. We'll provide an overview of program changes, introduce new Stage 2 criteria, discuss Stage 1 updates that impact your first two years of meaningful use, and offer insight about what's to come in the second stage of the program.

Part II:

BEYOND STAGE 1 MU

CHAPTER 6

Stage 2 Final Rules

Read more about the Stage 2 Final Rules and Stage 2 MU.

To get even more information about the second stage of the CMS EHR Incentive Programs, scan the QR code above or go to **stage2.theMUguide.com**.

In this chapter, we review the Stage 2 Final Rules, examine the regulations, and take a look at the requirements set forth for Stage 2 Meaningful Use.

Stage 2 Meaningful Use focuses on improving patient care and continues to deliver on the promise of achieving health and efficiency goals by (1) improving quality, safety, and efficiency while reducing health disparities, (2) engaging patients and families in their health care, (3) promoting and improve public and population health, (4) improving care coordination between providers, and (5) ensuring adequate privacy and security protections for personal health information.

A number of changes to the program, including, but not limited to, new criteria, changes to existing Stage 1 criteria, and programmatic updates, come with these final rules.

Overview

Under Stage 1 Meaningful Use, Medicare EPs are required to report against 15 Core Objectives and 5 out of 10 Menu Objectives, a total of 20 criteria, unless exclusions are met. Stage 2 Meaningful Use also contains 20 criteria, however, the distribution of those criteria differ from Stage 1.

In Stage 2, EPs are required to report against 17 Core Objectives and 3 out of 6 Menu Objectives, unless exclusions are met. In this second round of MU, new exclusion criteria have been introduced for new objectives and many Stage 1 exclusions carry over into Stage 2.

Eligibility Determination

There have been no fundamental changes in eligibility determination since program eligibility is determined by the Health Information and Technology for Economic and Clinical Health (HITECH) Act, which has not changed since its original publication. However, under regulatory purview of the incentive programs, CMS has instituted a change with respect to the definition of "Hospital-based EP" via the CMS Stage 2 Final Rule. According to CMS, if "EPs can demonstrate that they fund the acquisition, implementation, and maintenance of CEHRT, including supporting hardware, and interfaces needed for meaningful use without reimbursement from an eligible hospital or CAH—in lieu of using the hospital's CEHRT—can be determined non-hospital-based and potentially receive an incentive payment."

Note: Non-hospital-based EP determination will be made through an application process.

Timeline Changes

Under provisions of the CMS Stage 1 Final Rule, health care providers were originally required to advance to Stage 2 Meaningful Use after successfully meeting Stage 1 criteria for two years. However, the delayed onset of this second round of meaningful use has setback Stage 2 for Medicare EPs until 2014. As a result, EPs that started meaningful use in 2011 will complete three years of Stage 1 before proceeding to Stage 2. And, EPs starting meaningful use in 2012, and beyond, will complete two years of Stage 1 before proceeding to Stage 2.

Payment Adjustments for Non-compliance

Per the HITECH Act, Medicare EPs are subject to payment adjustments if they fail to satisfy meaningful use requirements before the program deadlines that go into effect beginning in 2015. Penalties in 2015, and beyond, will depend on individual EP meaningful use compliance two years before the year of payment adjustment. The following table outlines potential physician fee schedule adjustments based on program participation rates and calendar year.

POTENTIAL PAYMENT REDUCTIONS UNDER MEDICARE EHR INCENTIVE PROGRAM

Calendar Year	*Payment Reductions*
2015	Minus 1% of total Medicare fee schedule compensation
2016	Minus 2% of total Medicare fee schedule compensation
2017	Minus 3% of total Medicare fee schedule compensation
2018	Minus 3%, or minus 4% if >75% of EPs are not demonstrating meaningful use
2019+	Minus 3%, or minus 5% if >75% of EPs are not demonstrating meaningful use

Source: Centers for Medicare and Medicaid Services.

Note: EPs must demonstrate meaningful use annually in order to avoid payment adjustments in subsequent years.

EP Hardship Exceptions

To temporarily avoid payment adjustments for non-compliance, Medicare EPs may apply for hardship exceptions in one of four categories. EP hardship exceptions include:

- **Category I: Infrastructure**—EPs must demonstrate that they are in an area without sufficient Internet access or face insurmountable barriers to obtaining infrastructure.
- **Category II: New EPs**—Newly practicing EPs who would not have had time to become meaningful users can apply for a 2-year limited exception to payment adjustments.
- **Category III: Unforeseen Circumstances**—Examples may include a natural disaster or other unforeseeable barrier.

- **Category IV: Specialist/Provider**—EPs must demonstrate that they meet all three of the following criteria: (1) Lack of face-to-face or telemedicine interaction with patients (2) Lack of follow-up need with patients (3) Lack of control over the availability of CEHRT at their practice location (EPs who practice at multiple locations may be granted a hardship exception solely for lack of control over the availability of CEHRT).

Despite these exceptions, CMS does encourage EPs to comply with program requirements and obtain incentives for participation. And, EPs must apply for hardship exceptions no later than July 1 of the year before a payment adjustment year in order to avoid payment adjustments.

Note: Hardship exceptions will only be granted under specific circumstances and if CMS determines that providers have demonstrated that those circumstances pose a significant barrier to achieving meaningful use. CMS may also make regulatory changes that would eliminate the need for the exceptions in the future. Furthermore, EPs cannot be awarded hardship exceptions for more than 5 years total due to statutory limits. For more information about hardship exceptions and how to apply, go to **hardship.theMUguide.com**.

Stage 2 Meaningful Use Criteria for EPs

Even though Stage 2 Meaningful Use doesn't go into effect until you've successfully completed two years of Stage 1, it is important to have at least a basic understanding of what's to come in the next round of the program. Since many of the Stage 2 criteria are an evolution of Stage 1 criteria, knowing what Stage 2 has in store will assist you during your meaningful use planning.

At a high level, Stage 2 Meaningful Use requires Medicare EPs to report 17 Core Objectives and 3 out of 6 Menu Objectives, unless exclusions are met. Below you'll find a list of the criteria that were finalized for the second stage of the program.

STAGE 2 CORE SET

- **USE CPOE FOR ORDERS:** Use CPOE for **more than 60%** of medication, **30%** of laboratory, and **30%** of radiology orders (Stage 1 origin CORE 1, see page 44).
- **E-PRESCRIBING: More than 50%** of prescriptions written by the EP are queried for a drug formulary and transmitted electronically using CEHRT (Stage 1 origin CORE 4, see page 50; MENU 1, see page 78).
- **RECORD DEMOGRAPHICS:** Record demographics for **more than 80%** of all unique patients seen during the EHR reporting period (Stage 1 origin CORE 7, see page 56).
- **RECORD AND CHART VITAL SIGNS:** Record vital signs for **more than 80%** of all unique patients seen during the EHR reporting period (Stage 1 origin CORE 8, see page 58).
- **RECORD SMOKING STATUS:** Record smoking status for **more than 80%** of all unique patients 13 years old and older seen during the EHR reporting period (Stage 1 origin CORE 9, see page 60).
- **IMPLEMENT CLINICAL DECISION SUPPORT:** Implement **5 clinical decision support interventions** plus **drug-drug and drug-allergy interaction checks** (Stage 1 origin CORE 2, see page 46; CORE 11, see page 64).
- **INCORPORATE LAB TEST RESULTS:** Incorporate lab results for **more than 55%** of all clinical lab test results ordered during the EHR reporting period (Stage 1 origin MENU 2, see page 80).
- **GENERATE LISTS OF PATIENTS WITH SPECIFIC CONDITIONS:** Generate **at least one report** listing patients with a specific condition (Stage 1 origin MENU 3, see page 82).
- **PREVENTATIVE REMINDERS:** Provide reminders for preventive/follow-up care for **more than 10%** of patients with two or more office visits in the last 2 years (Stage 1 origin MENU 4, see page 84).
- **PATIENT ACCESS TO ONLINE HEALTH INFORMATION:** Provide online access to health information for **more than 50%** of all unique patients seen during the EHR reporting period with **more than 5%** actually accessing it (Stage 1 origin CORE 12, see page 66; MENU 5, see page 86).
- **PROVIDE CLINICAL SUMMARIES:** Provide office visit summaries within **1 business day for more than 50%** of office visits (Stage 1 origin CORE 13, see page 68).
- **PATIENT-SPECIFIC EDUCATION RESOURCES:** Provide education resources to **more than 10%** of all unique patients with office visits during the EHR reporting period (Stage 1 origin MENU 6, see page 88).
- **SECURE ELECTRONIC MESSAGES: More than 5%** of patients send secure messages to their EP (new in Stage 2).
- **MEDICATION RECONCILIATION:** Medication reconciliation at **more than 50%** of transitions of care (Stage 1 origin MENU 7, see page 90).
- **SUMMARY OF CARE RECORD FOR TRANSITIONS OF CARE OR REFERRAL:** Provide summary of care document for **more than 50%** of transitions of care and referrals **with 10% sent electronically** and **at least one sent to a recipient with a different EHR vendor or successfully testing with the CMS test EHR** (Stage 1 origin CORE 3, see page 48; CORE 5, see page 52; CORE 6, see page 54; MENU 8, see page 92).

- **CAPABILITY TO SUBMIT ELECTRONIC DATA TO IMMUNIZATION REGISTRIES:** Successful **ongoing transmission of immunization data** for the entire EHR reporting period (Stage 1 origin MENU 9, see page 94).
- **PROTECT ELECTRONIC HEALTH INFORMATION: Conduct or review security risk analysis** and incorporate in risk management process (Stage 1 origin CORE 15, see page 72).

STAGE 2 MENU SET

- **IMAGING RESULTS: More than 10%** of imaging results are accessible through CEHRT (new in Stage 2).
- **RECORD FAMILY HEALTH HISTORY:** Record family health history for **more than 20%** of all unique patients seen during the EHR reporting period (new in Stage 2).
- **CAPABILITY TO SUBMIT ELECTRONIC SYNDROMIC SUREILLANCE DATA:** Successful **ongoing transmission of syndromic surveillance data** for the entire EHR reporting period (Stage 1 origin MENU 10, see page 96).
- **IDENTIFY AND REPORT CANCER CASES:** Successful **ongoing transmission of cancer case information to a public health central cancer registry** for the entire EHR reporting period (new in Stage 2).
- **IDENTIFY AND REPORT SPECIFIC CASES:** Successful **ongoing transmission of specific case information to a specialized registry** for the entire EHR reporting period (new in Stage 2).
- **RECORD ELECTRONIC PROGRESS NOTES:** Enter an electronic progress note for **more than 30%** of unique patients with at least one office visit (new in Stage 2).

Note: Medicare EPs must select 3 out of 6 Menu Set criteria.

Batch Attestation

Prior to 2014, EPs must individually attest and report their data via the Medicare and Medicaid EHR Incentive Programs Registration and Attestation System. Under the CMS Stage 2 Final Rule, starting in 2014, groups are able to submit one attestation file for all of their individual EPs.

Certified EHR Technology (CEHRT)

The ONC 2014 Edition Standards & Certification Criteria Final Rule, which regulates the technology used by EPs for meaningful use compliance, was published in the *Federal Register*, along with the CMS Stage 2 Final Rule, on September 4, 2012. This final rule, which specifies the technical capabilities that EHR technology must include, introduced increased flexibility in the definition of certified EHR technology (CEHRT) with the goals of enhancing standards-based exchange, promoting EHR technology safety and security, enabling greater patient engagement, introducing greater transparency, and reducing regulatory burden.

Prior to 2014: 2011 Edition CEHRT

2011 Edition CEHRT can be used through 2013 to meet Stage 1 requirements. However, beginning in 2014, all providers participating in the program, regardless of stage, will need to implement and use 2014 Edition CEHRT.

> **Note:** EPs may use 2014 Edition CEHRT prior to 2014, but must report 2011 CQMs. Please refer to Chapter 3 for more information about CQMs.

2014+: 2014 Edition CEHRT

Starting in 2014, EPs must implement 2014 Edition CEHRT, regardless of program stage. Furthermore, this technology must be certified to meet the Base EHR definition as well as support core, menu, and CQM reporting requirements for the stage of meaningful use the EP is participating in.

- **Base EHR Definition:** Fundamental set of EHR capabilities certified against the 2014 Edition criteria that are universally applicable.
- **MU Core Definition:** Set of certified EHR capabilities an EP must have in order to satisfy core set objectives and measures they seek to achieve, unless an exclusion can be met.

- **MU Menu Definition:** Set of certified EHR capabilities an EP must have in order to satisfy menu set objectives and measures they seek to achieve.

Providers can choose to implement a 2014 Edition Complete EHR (technology certified to meet the Base EHR definition and all mandatory 2014 Edition criteria for the ambulatory setting) or 2014 Edition EHR Module(s) (single EHR Module, or combination of EHR Modules, certified to meet the 2014 Edition CEHRT definition).

In addition to the changes above, the ONC 2014 Edition Standards & Certification Criteria Final Rule introduced changes to the certification process. If your organization is seeking self-certification of EHR technology, it is important to take note of these program changes. Effective October 4, 2012, the Temporary Certification Program became permanent and was renamed the ONC HIT Certification Program. Under the new program, there have been revisions to EHR Module Certification requirements, application of new certification criteria to EHR technology, and price and test result transparency.

Stage 2 Final Rule Impact: For 2014 only, all providers, regardless of their stage of meaningful use, are only required to demonstrate MU for a 3-month EHR reporting period in order to provide adequate time for EPs to upgrade to 2014 Edition CEHRT, if needed.

Stay Up-to-Date: For the latest information about 2014 Edition CEHRT, go to **2014CEHRT.theMUguide.com**.

Part II:

BEYOND STAGE 1 MU

CHAPTER 7

Stage 2 Effects on Stage 1

Learn more about the effects of the Stage 2 Final Rules on Stage 1.

To review Stage 1 program changes and review specifications related to EPs, scan the QR code above or go to **effectsonstage1.theMUguide.com.**

In this chapter, we examine the impact of the Stage 2 Final Rules on Stage 1 Meaningful Use.

The release of the Stage 2 Final Rules brought about a number of changes to Stage 1 Meaningful Use. Many of these changes are optional beginning in 2013, but become mandatory in 2014 and beyond. Some Stage 1 criteria have been eliminated, or absorbed into the definition of meaningful use, while others have been updated to better align with program goals.

STAGE 1 CORE SET CHANGES

Stage 2 Final Rules have introduced specific changes to the following six (6) Stage 1 Core Set criteria.

- **42 CFR §495.6(d)(1):** Use computerized provider order entry (CPOE) for medication orders directly entered by any licensed health care professional who can enter orders into the medical record per state, local, and professional guidelines
  - **Alternate Measure (Stage 1 optional 2013+; effective Stage 2):** For details about Stage 1 changes related to this specific core set item, refer to page 44.
- **42 CFR §495.6(d)(4):** Generate and transmit permissible prescriptions electronically (eRx)
  - **Additional Exclusion (Stage 1 effective 2013+):** For details about Stage 1 changes related to this specific core set item, refer to page50.
- **42 CFR §495.6(d)(8):** Record and chart changes in vital signs: height, weight, blood pressure. Calculate and display BMI, plot and display growth charts for children 2–20 years (including BMI)
  - **Alternate Measure (Stage 1 optional 2013; effective 2014+):** For details about Stage 1 changes related to this specific core set item, refer to page 58.
  - **Alternate Exclusion (Stage 1 optional 2013; effective 2014+):** For details about Stage 1 changes related to this specific core set item, refer to page 58.
- **42 CFR §495.6(d)(10):** Report ambulatory clinical quality measures to CMS or the States
  - **Eliminated/Absorbed into MU Definition (Stage 1 effective 2013+):** For details about Stage 1 changes related to this specific core set item, refer to page 62.
- **42 CFR §495.6(d)(12):** Provide patients with an electronic copy of their health information (including diagnostic test results, problem list, medication list, medication allergies) upon request
  - **New Objective (replaces current criteria; Stage 1 effective 2014+):** For details about Stage 1 changes related to this specific core set item, refer to page 66.
  - **New Measure (replaces current criteria; Stage 1 effective 2014+):** For details about Stage 1 changes related to this specific core set item, refer to page 66.
- **42 CFR §495.6(d)(14):** Capability to exchange key clinical information (for example: problem list, medication list, medication allergies, diagnostic test results) among providers of care and patient-authorized entities electronically
  - **Eliminated (Stage 1 effective 2013+):** For details about Stage 1 changes related to this specific core set item, refer to page 70.

STAGE 1 MENU SET CHANGES

Stage 2 Final Rules have introduced specific changes to the following three (3) Stage 1 Menu Set criteria.

- **42 CFR §495.6(e)(5):** Provide patients with timely electronic access to their health information (including lab results, problem list, medication lists, medication allergies) within four business days of the information being available to the EP
  - **New Objective (replaces current criteria; moves to Core Set; Stage 1 effective 2014+):** For details about Stage 1 changes related to this specific menu set item, refer to page 86.
  - **New Measure (replaces current criteria; moves to Core Set; Stage 1 effective 2014+):** For details about Stage 1 changes related to this specific menu set item, refer to page 86.
- **42 CFR §495.6(e)(9):** Capability to submit electronic data to immunization registries or Immunization Information Systems and actual submission in accordance with applicable law and practice
  - **New Objective (replaces current criteria; Stage 1 effective 2013+):** For details about Stage 1 changes related to this specific menu set item, refer to page 94.
- **42 CFR §495.6(e)(10):** Capability to submit electronic syndromic surveillance data to public health agencies and actual submission in accordance with applicable law and practice
  - **New Objective (replaces current criteria; Stage 1 effective 2013+):** For details about Stage 1 changes related to this specific menu set item, refer to page 96.

Stage 2 Final Rule Impact: Prior to 2014, EPs can still claim exclusions (if applicable) and reduce their menu set reporting obligations. Beginning in 2014, EPs will not be allowed to lower their total menu set objectives based on menu set exclusions.

Clinical Quality Measure (CQM) Changes

Due to provisions in the CMS Stage 2 Final Rule, 42 CFR §495.6(d)(10) will no longer be a separate standalone objective beginning in 2013. 42 CFR §495.6(d)(10) has been incorporated directly into the definition of meaningful use, and as such, program participants are still required to report CQMs in order to achieve meaningful use. Prior to 2014, EPs are required to demonstrate and report a total of 6 out of 44 clinical quality measures (3 core/alternate core measures and 3 discretionary measures from the remaining 38 measures). Beginning in 2014, providers will be required to report against new CY2014 CQMs (refer to Chapter 3 for more information about CQMs).

Note: In 2012 and 2013, Stage 1 CQM reporting may be conducted via Attestation (**attestation.theMUguide.com**) or eReporting Pilot (**ereporting.theMUguide.com**). Starting in 2014, all Medicare EPs must submit CQM data via Attestation in their first year and, in subsequent years, must electronically submit CQM data to CMS.

Part III:

FAQs AND RESOURCES

In this final section, we take a look at frequently asked questions that relate to your initial years of program participation as well as offer additional resources to help you as you embark on your meaningful use journey.

Part III:

FAQs AND RESOURCES

CHAPTER 8

Frequently Asked Questions

Read the most current FAQs online.

As with any government program that changes over time, so do the frequently asked questions. To view the most current list of FAQs that are relevant to EPs in their first two years, scan the QR code above or go to **first2yearfaqs.theMUguide.com**.

In this chapter, we address some of the most common questions about meaningful use as they relate to your first two years of the program—this compilation of FAQs has been collected in part from the government program websites.

CMS FAQ#2791:
CEHRT POSSESSION AND REGISTRATION

Question: Do I need to have an electronic health record (EHR) system in order to register for the Medicare and Medicaid EHR Incentive Programs?

Answer: You do not need to have a certified EHR in order to register for the Medicare and Medicaid EHR Incentive Programs. However, to receive an incentive payment under the Medicare program, you must attest that you have demonstrated meaningful use of certified EHR technology (CEHRT) during the EHR reporting period. For the first year of payment, the EHR reporting period is 90 consecutive days within the calendar year for eligible professionals (EPs) or within the Federal fiscal year for eligible hospitals and critical access hospitals (CAHs).

With regard to the Medicaid EHR Incentive Program, for the first year of payment, EPs and hospitals must have adopted, implemented, upgraded certified EHR technology before they can receive an EHR incentive payment from the State. As an alternative to demonstrating that they have adopted, implemented or upgraded certified EHR technology, for the first year of payment, the EP or hospital may demonstrate that they are meaningful users of certified EHR technology for the 90-day EHR reporting period.

CMS FAQ#2861:
PROGRAM REGISTRATION

Question: Do providers register only once for the Medicare and Medicaid Electronic Health Record (EHR) Incentive Programs, or must they register every year?

Answer: Providers are only required to register once for the Medicare and Medicaid EHR Incentive Programs. However, they must successfully demonstrate that they have either adopted, implemented or upgraded (first participation year for Medicaid) or meaningfully used certified EHR technology each year in order to receive an incentive payment for that year. Additionally, providers seeking the Medicaid incentive must annually re-attest to other program requirements, such as meeting the required patient volume thresholds. Providers will register using the Medicare and Medicaid EHR Incentive Program Registration & Attestation System, a web- based system. Providers who have elected to participate in the Medicare EHR Incentive Program will also use this system to attest to their program eligibility and meaningful use. Providers who select the Medicaid EHR Incentive Program will demonstrate their eligibility and attest via their State Medicaid Agency's system. If any basic registration information changes, the provider will need to update their information in the Medicare and Medicaid EHR Incentive Program.

CMS FAQ#2621:
PARTICIPATING IN BOTH (MEDICARE AND MEDICAID VERSION) PROGRAMS

Question: Can eligible professionals (EPs) receive electronic health record (EHR) incentive payments from both the Medicare and Medicaid programs?

Answer: Not for the same year. If an EP meets the requirements of both programs, they must choose to receive an EHR incentive payment under either the Medicare program or the Medicaid program. After a payment has been made, the EP may only switch programs once before 2015.

CMS FAQ#2859:
INCENTIVE PAYMENT TAX TREATMENT

Question: Are payments from the Medicare and Medicaid Electronic Health Record (EHR) Incentive Programs subject to federal income tax?

Answer: We note that nothing in the Act excludes such payments from taxation or as tax-free income. Therefore, it is our belief that incentive payments would be treated like any other income. Providers should consult with a tax advisor or the Internal Revenue Service regarding how to properly report this income on their filings.

CMS FAQ#2879:
EPs PRACTICING AT ACADEMIC MEDICAL CENTERS

Question: Will academic physicians employed by an academic medical center billing under the same CMS facility number as the hospital be allowed to participate as eligible professionals (EPs) in the Medicare and Medicaid Electronic Health Record (EHR) Incentive Programs if they qualify in all other aspects?

Answer: Physicians who furnish substantially all, defined as 90% or more, of their covered professional services in either an inpatient (POS 21) or emergency department (POS 23) of a hospital are considered to be hospital-based and are therefore not eligible for incentive payments under the Medicare and Medicaid EHR Incentive Programs. If an academic physician is employed by an academic medical center, bills under the same CMS Certification Number (CCN), and is considered hospital-based according to the definition above, then the academic physician would not be eligible to participate as an eligible professional in the Medicare and Medicaid EHR Incentive Programs.

CMS FAQ#2805:
SPECIAL INCENTIVES FOR RURAL PROVIDERS

Question: Are there any special incentives for rural providers in the Medicare and Medicare Electronic Health Record (EHR) Incentive Programs?

Answer: Under the Medicare EHR Incentive Program, the maximum allowed charge threshold for the annual incentive payment limit for each payment year will be increased by 10 percent for eligible professionals (EPs) who predominantly furnish services in a rural or urban geographic Health Professional Shortage Area (HPSA). Critical access hospitals (CAHs) can receive an incentive payment amount equal to the product of its reasonable costs incurred for the purchase of certified EHR technology and the Medicare share percentage. Under the Medicaid EHR Incentive Program, there are no additional incentives for rural providers, beyond the incentives already available.

CMS FAQ#2901:
INCENTIVE PAYMENT TERMS

Question: After successfully demonstrating meaningful use for the Medicare and Medicaid Electronic Health Record (EHR) Incentive Program, will incentive payments be paid as a lump sum or in multiple installments?

Answer: Eligible professionals (EPs) participating in the Medicare EHR Incentive Program will receive a single lump sum payment for each year they successfully demonstrate meaningful use of certified EHR technology. Eligible hospitals and critical access hospitals (CAHs) participating in the Medicare EHR Incentive Program will first receive an initial payment. The final payment will be determined at the time of settling the hospital cost report. Payments to Medicare providers will be made to the taxpayer identification number (TIN) selected at the time of registration, through the same channels their claims payments are made. However, for EPs practicing in a health professional shortage area (HPSA), the additional incentive payment will be paid separately to the same TIN as the incentive payment.

Medicaid incentives will be paid by the States. EPs, eligible hospitals, and CAHs participating in the Medicaid EHR Incentive Program should check with their State.

CMS FAQ#2883:
SCOPE OF PRACTICE EXCLUSIONS

Question: If an eligible professional (EP) is unable to meet the measure of a meaningful use objective because it is outside of the scope of his or her practice, will the EP be excluded from meeting the measure of that objective under the Medicare and Medicaid Electronic Health Record (EHR) Incentive Programs?

Answer: Some meaningful use objectives provide exclusions and others do not. Exclusions are available only when our regulations specifically provide for an exclusion. EPs may be excluded from meeting an objective if they meet the circumstances of the exclusion. If an EP is unable to meet a meaningful use objective for which no exclusion is available, then that EP would not be able to successfully demonstrate meaningful use and would not receive incentive payments under the Medicare and Medicaid EHR Incentive Programs.

CMS FAQ#3069:
SPECIALTY PROVIDERS

Question: Do specialty providers have to meet all of the meaningful use objectives for the Medicare and Medicaid EHR Incentive Programs, or can they ignore the objectives that are not relevant to their scope of practice?

Answer: For eligible professionals (EPs) who participate in the Medicare and Medicaid EHR Incentive Programs, there are a total of 25 meaningful use objectives. To qualify for an incentive payment, 20 of these 25 objectives must be met. There are 15 required core objectives. The remaining 5 objectives may be chosen from the list of 10 menu set objectives. Certain objectives do provide exclusions. If an EP meets the criteria for that exclusion, then the EP can claim that exclusion during attestation. However, if an exclusion is not provided, or if the EP does not meet the criteria for an existing exclusion, then the EP must meet the measure of the objective in order to successfully demonstrate meaningful use and receive an EHR incentive payment. Failure to meet the measure of an objective or to qualify for an exclusion for the objective will prevent an EP from successfully demonstrating meaningful use and receiving an incentive payment.

CMS FAQ#3609:
MULTIPLE PRACTICE LOCATIONS

Question: For the Medicare and Medicaid Electronic Health Record (EHR) Incentive Programs, how should an eligible professional (EP), eligible hospital, or critical access hospital (CAH) that sees patients in multiple practice locations equipped with certified EHR technology calculate numerators and denominators for the meaningful use objectives and measures?

Answer: EPs, eligible hospitals, and CAHs should look at the measure of each meaningful use objective to determine the appropriate calculation method for individual numerators and denominators. The calculation of the numerator and denominator for each measure is explained in the July 28, 2010 Final Rule (75 FR 44314).

For objectives that require a simple count of actions (e.g., number of permissible prescriptions written, for the objective of "Generate and transmit permissible prescriptions electronically (eRx)"; number of patient requests for an electronic copy of their health information, for the objective of "Provide patients with an electronic copy of their health information"; etc.), EPs, eligible hospitals, and CAHs can add the numerators and denominators calculated by each certified EHR system in order to arrive at an accurate total for the numerator and denominator of the measure.

For objectives that require an action to be taken on behalf of a percentage of "unique patients" (e.g., the objectives of "Record demographics", "Record vital signs", etc.), EPs, eligible hospitals, and CAHs may also add the numerators and denominators calculated by each certified EHR system in order to arrive at an accurate total for the numerator and denominator of the measure. Previously, CMS had advised providers to reconcile information so that they only reported unique patients. However, because it is not possible for providers to increase their overall percentage of actions taken by adding numerators and denominators from multiple systems, we now permit simple addition for all meaningful use objectives.

Please keep in mind that patients whose records are not maintained in certified EHR technology will need to be added to denominators whenever applicable in order to provide accurate numbers.

To report clinical quality measures, EPs who practice in multiple locations that are equipped with certified EHR technology should generate a report from each of those certified EHR systems and then add the numerators, denominators, and exclusions from each generated report in order to arrive at a number that reflects the total data output for patient encounters at those locations. To report clinical quality measures, eligible hospitals and CAHs that have multiple systems should generate a report from each of those certified EHR systems and then add the numerators, denominators, and exclusions from each generated report in order to arrive at a number that reflects the total data output for patient encounters in the relevant departments of the eligible hospital or CAH (e.g., inpatient or emergency department (POS 21 or 23)).

ADDITIONAL FAQs

CMS Regulations FAQ Website: The official CMS FAQ website offers detailed answers to the most frequently asked CMS-related questions. Go to **cmsfaqs.theMUguide.com**.

ONC Regulations FAQ Website: The official ONC FAQ website offers detailed answers to the most frequently asked ONC-related questions. Go to **oncfaqs.theMUguide.com**.

Part III:

FAQs AND RESOURCES

CHAPTER 9

Resources and Tools

Take advantage of available resources and tools.

To view the most recent list of resources that will help you on your path to meaningful use, scan the QR code above or go to **resources.theMUguide.com**.

In this chapter, we further prepare you for your first two years of meaningful use by taking a look at resources to help you along the way.

Meaningful use success begins with understanding the program fundamentals. Whether that means visiting the government program website, going to lectures, reading articles, listening to podcasts, attending tradeshows, or reading the thousands of pages of regulations, it is imperative that you understand the fundamentals of the CMS EHR Incentive Programs and what they mean to your health care practice. We recommend you use the following resources to better understand the fundamentals of meaningful use and better prepare for your first two years of participation.

GETTING STARTED

While there are many resources available online with information about the CMS EHR Incentive Programs, these resources are a great start for those beginning their meaningful use journey.

CMS EHR Incentive Programs Eligibility: CMS has numerous resources available on the EHR Incentive Programs website, including eligibility flowcharts and interactive eligibility tools to help get you started. Go to **cmseligibilitychart.theMUguide.com** and **cmseligibilitytool.theMUguide.com** to access these resources.

MU Flowchart (DoYouMU.com): This website offers eligible professionals (EPs) an online guide that steps through an organized process to determine your best methods for participation. Go to **DoYouMU.com**.

FEDERAL RESOURCES

These federal resources provide a wealth of information about meaningful use legislation, regulations, and program requirements.

CMS Medicare and Medicaid Electronic Heath Records (EHR) Incentive Programs Website: The official website for the CMS EHR Incentive Programs with information and program details, registration links, attestation links, FAQs, and more. Go to **cms.theMUguide.com**.

The Office of the National Coordinator (ONC) for Health Information Technology: The official website for the ONC. Go to **onc.theMUguide.com**.

CMS EHR Incentive Programs Listserv: Another great resource is the CMS EHR Incentive Programs Listserv, which offers timely, authoritative information about the government program. Through this system, CMS keeps EPs informed about upcoming deadlines, answers questions and addresses concerns about the program, circulates updates, and notifies subscribers of new FAQ documents related to the incentive programs. To subscribe to the CMS EHR Incentive Programs Listserv, go to **ehrlistserv.theMUguide.com**.

Medicare and Medicaid Programs Electronic Health Record Incentive Program Final Rule: This Final Rule implements the provisions of the American Recovery and Reinvestment Act (ARRA) of 2009 (Pub. L. 111-5) that provide incentive payments to eligible professionals (EPs), eligible hospitals (EHs), and critical access hospitals (CAHs) participating in Medicare and Medicaid programs that adopt and successfully demonstrate meaningful use of certified electronic health record (EHR) technology. This document specifies the initial criteria EPs, EHs, and CAHs must meet in order to qualify for an incentive payment, calculation of the incentive payment amounts, payment adjustments under Medicare for covered professional services and inpatient hospital services provided by EPs, EHs, and CAHs failing to demonstrate meaningful use of certified EHR technology, and other program participation requirements. Go to **cmsfinalrule.theMUguide.com**.

Medicare and Medicaid Programs Electronic Health Record Incentive Program Final Rule—Stage 2: This final rule specifies the Stage 2 criteria that eligible professionals (EPs), eligible hospitals, and critical access hospitals (CAHs) must meet in order to qualify for Medicare and/or Medicaid electronic health record (EHR) incentive payments. In addition, it specifies payment adjustments under Medicare for covered professional services and hospital services provided by EPs, eligible hospitals, and CAHs failing to demonstrate meaningful use of certified EHR technology (CEHRT) and other program participation requirements. This final rule revises certain Stage 1 criteria, as finalized in the July 28, 2010 Final Rule, as well as criteria that apply regardless of Stage. Go to **cmsfinalrule2.theMUguide.com**.

Health Information Technology Initial Set of Standards, Implementation Specifications, and Certification Criteria for Electronic Health Record Technology Final Rule: This document fully outlines the initial set of standards, implementation specifications, and certification criteria to ensure alignment with final Stage 1 Meaningful Use objectives and measures. Go to **oncfinalrule.theMUguide.com**.

Health Information Technology Initial Set of Standards, Implementation Specifications, and Certification Criteria for Electronic Health Record Technology, 2014 Edition; Revisions to the Permanent Certification Program for Health Information Technology: With this final rule, the Secretary of Health and Human Services adopts certification criteria that establish the technical capabilities and specify the related standards and implementation specifications that CEHRT will need to include to, at a minimum, support the achievement of meaningful use by eligible professionals, eligible hospitals, and critical access hospitals under the Medicare and Medicaid EHR Incentive Programs beginning with the EHR reporting periods in fiscal year and calendar year 2014. This final rule also makes changes to the permanent certification program for health information technology, including changing the program's name to the ONC HIT Certification Program. Go to **oncfinalrule2014.theMUguide.com**.

Certified HIT Product List (CHPL): This official program website provides the authoritative, comprehensive listing of Complete EHRs and EHR Modules that have been tested and certified under the certification program maintained by the Office of the National Coordinator for Health IT (ONC). Each CEHRT listed on this website has been certified by an ONC-Authorized Testing and Certification Body (ONC-ATCB) and reported to the ONC. Go to **chpl.theMUguide.com**.

Regional Extension Centers (RECs): Regional Extension Centers (RECs) were created in 2009 under the HITECH Act and finalized in September 2010. Under the HITECH Act, $677 million was allocated to support the nationwide system of 62 RECs. RECs help physicians, clinics, and hospitals move from paper-based medical records to EHRs. These organizations target their assistance to eligible primary care providers in smaller practices as well as small and rural hospitals and public health clinics. They also serve as resources for all providers in a given geographic region. The performance of each REC will be evaluated every two years to determine if continued federal support for the center is in the best interest of the extension program. Go to **recs.theMUguide.com**.

PROGRAM FACTS SHEETS

The official program fact sheets found on these government websites offer concise overviews and detailed information about the incentive programs.

Electronic Health Records at a Glance: This fact sheet provides a concise overview of EHRs and answers such questions as why EHRs are held to meaningful use requirements, and provides a look ahead with timetables and an outline of the incentive programs. Go to **ataglance.theMUguide.com**.

CMS and ONC Final Regulations Define Meaningful Use and Set Standards for Electronic Health Record Incentive Program: This fact sheet discusses the CMS Final Rule, the ONC Final Rule, timetable for implementation, the meaningful use model, the approach to supporting EHR adoption, key provisions of the final rules, and insight into the development of the rules. Go to **definetheprogram.theMUguide.com**.

CMS Finalized Definition of Meaningful Use of Certified Electronic Health Records (EHR) Technology: This fact sheet defines meaningful use policy goals, reviews the development of Stage 1 criteria, and discusses policy goals beyond Stage 1 Meaningful Use. Go to **definecertified.theMUguide.com**.

CMS Medicare and Medicaid EHR Incentive Programs: Stage 2 Final Rule Fact Sheet: This fact sheet provides highlights of the CMS Stage 2 Final Rule. Go to **cmsfactsheet2.theMUguide.com**.

ONC Fact Sheet: 2014 Edition Standards & Certification Criteria Final Rule: This fact sheet provides highlights of the ONC 2014 Edition Standards & Certification Criteria Final Rule. Go to **oncfactsheet2014.theMUguide.com**.

MU-RELATED BLOGS AND SOCIAL MEDIA

There are a few official government blogs as well as social media resources, such as Twitter, that offer valuable information and updates about meaningful use.

Health IT Buzz Blog: This blog is a service of the ONC and was created to answer questions and create a conversation about the challenges and successes health care providers and organizations are experiencing as they transition to Electronic Health Records. Go to **hitblog.theMUguide.com**.

Federal Advisory Committee Blog:
Go to **facblog.theMUguide.com**.

Twitter: Social media outlets such as Twitter are a fantastic resource for up-to-the-minute news, announcements, and updates related to meaningful use. To find MU-related content, we recommend searching with the following hashtags:

#MEANINGFULUSE	**#STAGE2**	**#HITECH**
#MU	**#STAGE2MU**	**#EHR**
#STAGE1	**#STAGE3**	**#CMS**
#STAGE1MU	**#STAGE3MU**	**#ONC**

Appendix

With thousands of pages of regulations, the CMS EHR Incentive Programs documentation has introduced dozens of new acronyms. While not fully comprehensive, the list below outlines the common acronyms used throughout this guide and meaningful use literature.

ACO Accountable Care Organizations

ANSI American National Standards Institute

ARRA American Recovery and Reinvestment Act of 2009

CAH Critical Access Hospital

CCR Continuity of Care Record

CDA Clinical Document Architecture

CDC Centers for Disease Control and Prevention

CEHRT Certified Electronic Health Record Technology *(pronounced "cert")*

CFR Code of Federal Regulations

CHPL Certified Health IT Product List

CMS Centers for Medicare & Medicaid Services

CPOE Computerized Physician (or Provider) Order Entry

CQM Clinical Quality Measures

EH Eligible Hospital

EHR Electronic Health Record

EMR Electronic Medical Record

EP Eligible Professional

FACA Federal Advisory Committee Act

FFS Fee-for-Service

HHS U.S. Department of Health and Human Services

HIE Health Information Exchange

HIPAA Health Insurance Portability and Accountability Act

HIT Health Information Technology

HITECH Health Information Technology for Economic and Clinical Health

HITRC Healthcare Information Technology Research Center

HITSP Healthcare Information Technology Standards Panel

HL7 Health Level Seven

HPSA Health Professional Shortage Area

ICD International Classification for Diseases

NIST National Institute of Standards and Technology

NLM National Library of Medicine

NPI National Provider Identifier

NPPES National Plan and Provider Enumeration System

NPRM Notice of Proposed Rulemaking

NQF National Quality Forum

ONC Office of the National Coordinator for Health Information Technology

PECOS Provider Enrollment, Chain, and Ownership System

PQRI Physician Quality Reporting Initiative

PQRS Physician Quality Reporting System

REC Regional Extension Center

XML Extensible Markup Language

Medicare and Medicaid Programs; Electronic Health Record Incentive Program. Comparison of Meaningful Use Objectives Between the Proposed Rule to the Final Rule. 13 July 2010. Web.

U.S. Department of Commerce. The National Institute of Standards and Technology. Health Information Technology. Standards and Testing. Meaningful Use Test Method. Web. <http://www.nist.gov/healthcare/testing/ mutestmethod.cfm/>.

U.S. Department of Health and Human Services. Centers for Medicare & Medicaid Services. CMS EHR Incentive Programs Official Website. Web. <http:// www.cms.gov/ehrincentiveprograms/>.

U.S. Department of Health and Human Services. Centers for Medicare & Medicaid Services.

U.S. Department of Health and Human Services. Centers for Medicare & Medicaid Services. Medicare and Medicaid Programs; Electronic Health Record Incentive Program. Final Rule. 42 CFR Parts 412, 413, 422, and 495. 28 July 2010. Print.

U.S. Department of Health and Human Services. Centers for Medicare & Medicaid Services. Medicare and Medicaid Programs; Electronic Health Record Incentive Program: Stage 2. Final Rule. 42 CFR Parts 412, 413, and 495. 4 September 2012. Print.

U.S. Department of Health and Human Services. Office of the National Coordinator for Health Information Technology. Certified Health IT Product List. Web. <http://oncchpl.force.com/ehrcert>.

U.S. Department of Health and Human Services. Office of the National Coordinator for Health Information Technology. Establishment of the Temporary Certification Program for Health Information Technology. Part II. Final Rule. 42 CFR Part 170. 24 June 2010. Print.

U.S. Department of Health and Human Services. Office of the National Coordinator for Health Information Technology. Federal Advisory Committee Blog. Web. <http://healthit.hhs.gov/blog/faca/>.

U.S. Department of Health and Human Services. Office of the National Coordinator for Health Information Technology. Health Information Technology: Initial Set of Standards, Implementation Specifications, and Certification Criteria for Electronic Health Record Technology. Part III. Final Rule. 42 CFR Part 170. 28 July 2010. Print.

U.S. Department of Health and Human Services. Office of the National Coordinator for Health Information Technology. Health Information Technology: Initial Set of Standards, Implementation Specifications, and Certification Criteria for Electronic Health Record Technology. Interim Final Rule. 42 CFR Part 170. 13 January 2010. Print.

U.S. Department of Health and Human Services. Office of the National Coordinator for Health Information Technology. Health Information Technology: Initial Set of Standards, Implementation Specifications, and Certification Criteria for Electronic Health Record Technology, 2014 Edition; Revisions to the Permanent Certification Program for Health Information Technology. Final Rule. 42 CFR Part 170. 4 September 2012. Print.

U.S. Department of Health and Human Services. Office of the National Coordinator for Health Information Technology. HealthITBuzz Blog. Web. <http://www.healthit.gov/buzz-blog/>.

U.S. Department of Health and Human Services. Office of the National Coordinator for Health Information Technology. Regulations and Guidance. Electronic Health Records and Meaningful Use. Web. <http://healthit.hhs.gov/ portal/server.pt?open=512&objID=2996&mode=2>.

About the authors

Jonathon L. Dreyer is a senior health care marketing professional in Boston, Massachusetts. His deep understanding of medical imaging technology and healthcare IT has contributed to the development and successful deployment of technology across a number of health care verticals. He has authored several articles on clinical decision support, radiology reporting, speech recognition, business intelligence, electronic health records, meaningful use, and mHealth, and is an active blogger and contributor to standards and interoperability projects.

Keith J. Dreyer, DO, PhD, FACR, FSIIM is the Vice Chairman of Radiology Informatics at Massachusetts General Hospital and Assistant Professor of Radiology at the Harvard Medical School. He is a Diagnostic Specialist, certified by the American Board of Radiology with a PhD in Computer Science. Dr. Dreyer holds, and has held, numerous board and committee positions with the ACR, RSNA, SIIM, and other national medical societies, and has authored numerous scientific papers, articles, and books, as well as lectures worldwide on digital imaging, medical informatics, clinical language understanding, and electronic health records.

50765731R00099

Made in the USA
Lexington, KY
29 March 2016